PERSONAL AGGRESSIVENESS
AND WAR

Founded by C. K. Ogden

The International Library of Psychology

SOCIAL PSYCHOLOGY
In 7 Volumes

PERSONAL
AGGRESSIVENESS AND WAR

E F M DURBIN AND JOHN BOWLBY

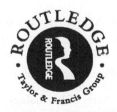

First published in 1949
by Routledge

Reprinted in 1999, 2000, 2001
by Routledge
2 Park Square, Milton Park, Abingdon, Oxfordshire OX14 4RN
711 Third Avenue, New York, NY 10017
First issued in paperback 2014

Routledge is an imprint of the Taylor and Francis Group, an informa company

Transferred to Digital Printing 2007

British Library Cataloguing in Publication Data
A CIP catalogue record for this book
is available from the British Library

Personal Aggressiveness and War
ISBN 978-0-415-21116-1 (hbk)
ISBN 978-0-415-75816-1 (pbk)

Social Psychology: 7 Volumes
ISBN 978-0-415-21134-5
The International Library of Psychology: 204 Volumes
ISBN 978-0-415-19132-6

PREFACE

THIS essay appeared originally in 1938 as part of a symposium entitled *War and Democracy* edited by E. F. M. Durbin and G. E. G. Catlin. The decision to publish it separately has been taken because it was felt that it possessed a certain unity in itself and might have some value as an introduction to the scientific study of the causes of fighting and war.

We would like, however, to take this opportunity to correct a misunderstanding of our aims that has already arisen. We make no claim to explain the origins of any particular war. In our view the causes of any specific war are complex and their analysis must remain the task of the historian. Our attempt has been rather to describe and analyse the general psychological forces lying behind the timeless and ubiquitous urge to fight and kill. Just as it is the task of the physicist to study the general laws governing the behaviour of forces, such as electricity or gravitation, and of others, the astronomer or engineer, to study their particular manifestations, so do we conceive it to be the task of the social psychologist to isolate and understand the instinctive forces lying behind all human conduct, whilst the historian explains how these forces come to express themselves in a specific sequence of events.

Some confusion has also arisen over our use of the term 'animism.' On reflection it seems to us that 'personalism' would be a better term since it has not been used for other purposes and is an appropriate description of the phenomena in question. Some technical and specific term is clearly needed to describe the tendency—common in the human mind—to attribute all events to the agency of some deliberate will.

A word of explanation is required for the eccentric arrangement of the present work. In order to balance the original

v

symposium, a large part of this essay was made into an Appendix, a title that it still holds. It would, however, be more accurate if the first fifty pages were to be entitled Part I and the remainder Part II of the Book. In the first part one of us discusses the comparative merits of three theories of war, whilst in the second part an attempt is made to present some of the psychological evidence which underlies and justifies the psychological theories discussed in the first part.

Finally, we should like to point out that certain of the references to other parts of the book refer to essays in the original symposium, *War and Democracy*, published by Messrs. Kegan Paul, Trench, Trubner and Co., Ltd.

E. F. M. D.

February, 1939.   J. M. B.

TABLE OF CONTENTS

I

II

III

APPENDIX

An Examination of the Psychological and Anthropological Evidence

PERSONAL AGGRESSIVENESS AND WAR

I

THE purpose of this article is to examine the bearing of some recent biological and psychological work upon the theories of the cause of war.

The authors hold that war—or organized fighting between large groups of adult human beings—must be regarded as one species of a larger genus, the genus of *fighting*. Fighting is plainly a common, indeed a universal, form of human behaviour. It extends beyond the borders of humanity into the types of mammals most closely related in the evolutionary classification to the common ancestors of man and other apes. War between groups within the nation and between nations are obvious and important examples of this type of behaviour. Since this is so, it must of necessity follow that the simplest and most general causes of war are only to be found in the causes of fighting, just as the simplest and most general causes of falling downstairs are to be found in the causes of falling down.

Such a simple thesis could hardly be expected to contain any important conclusion. Yet if the causes of war are to be found in their simplest form only in phenomena more widely dispersed in space and time than comparatively recent forms of political and economic organization, like the nation State and the capitalist system, it must surely follow that theories tracing the cause of war either to ' capitalism ' or ' nationalism ' can only at the best contain part of the truth. Nevertheless, it is theories of this kind that are fashionable in the current discussions of the cause of war.

We shall revert at length to the bearing of our own views upon these theories. In the meantime, it is our primary task to examine some of the evidence recently collected on the extent and causes of fighting. The procedure that we propose to follow is to summarize and analyse the descriptive work that has been done upon fighting among apes, children, and civilized adults in the Appendix, and to use the conclusions

3

to be derived from that work in the argument of this article. The empirical evidence that is available is far from complete, but we think that it is more than sufficient to sustain a number of most important conclusions about the effective causes of war.

Fighting, as we have already pointed out, is a form of behaviour widely distributed through history and nature. It occurs in the form of group conflict throughout recorded time. It takes place spasmodically between individuals in civilized countries. It occurs among primitives, among children, and among apes. Whether one looks back through time or downwards to simpler forms of social organization, it is a common practice for individuals or groups to seek to change their environment by force, and for other individuals and groups to meet force with force.

But fighting, or the appeal to force, while universal in distribution, is not continuous in time. The most warlike groups and the most aggressive individuals spend considerable periods in peaceful toleration of, and positive co-operation with, other animals or persons. Most organized communities have enjoyed longer periods of peace than of war. The greater part of human activity—of man-hours—is spent, not in war, but in peaceful co-operation. The scientific problem is, therefore, twofold—why is there peaceful co-operation and why does peaceful co-operation sometimes break down into war? The practical problem—at least, for lovers of peace— is how peaceful co-operation is to be preserved against the universal tendency exhibited in history for it to degenerate into war.

PEACEFUL CO-OPERATION

What, then, are the simplest causes of peaceful co-opera- tion? Here it is necessary to distinguish between groups with and without ' government '—that is, an apparatus of force constructed with the conscious and explicit purpose of preserving peace within the group. Clearly, the existence of a powerful organization taking action to preserve peace itself constitutes a strong and immediate cause for the appearance of peace.[1] With the consequence of this obvious point we shall

---

[1] We feel unable to accept Dr. Glover's rather casual rejection of instruments of government and collective security as a means of preserving peace. (See

be concerned at the end of this article. For the moment, however, we are interested in a prior and more fundamental question. What are the causes of peace in a group without government or any effective machinery for the restraint of fighting ? Why do animals co-operate in the absence of any agent powerful enough to prevent them from fighting ?

Now a survey of the life of mammals in general, and of apes and men in particular,[1] suggests that the causes of peace in the absence of government are, for the extra-familial group,[2] of three main kinds :

1. The obvious, most important, and overwhelming advantage to be derived from peace lies in the division of labour and the possibility of thus achieving purposes desired by the individual but obtainable only by active co-operation with others. This is so plain in the case of adult human society that the point is scarcely worth elaborating. The whole of the difference in the variety of satisfactions open to the individual in isolation and the same person in the active membership of a peaceful society, measures the advantages to be derived from continuous co-operation between adults. The extent of co-operation in any groups other than adult human societies is, of course, much more limited. But groups of children co-operate in simple tasks and in games that require a specialization of function between the individual members of the group. And there is some evidence to suggest that apes exhibit still simpler forms of co-operation and that even mammals who hunt and live in herds develop simple differentiation of function for various common purposes of defence or attack[3].

Co-operation extends enormously the opportunities for life and satisfaction within groups that have developed it. It

Glover, *The Dangers of being Human*.) We feel that he does not appreciate the strength of the will to co-operate expressed in them. We shall consider this point at some length at the end of Part III of this article.

[1] See Appendix *passim*.

[2] We have not concerned ourselves with the reasons for peace within the family, (*a*) because it leads at once to the rather different question of the nature of sexual and familial ties ; (*b*) because the family usually exhibits the phenomenon of patriarchal and matriarchal authority.

[3] This last point is not universally conceded by the students of animal behaviour. Apes appear to scratch each other and some herds of herbivores seem to maintain a system of outposts and sentries. But it has been denied that these phenomena can be compared with the purposive co-operation found in human society. The conflict of view could only be resolved by further investigation.

is reasonable to presume that these advantages are also *causes* of co-operation, since many of the results of co-operation are of survival value. In any case, few persons would wish to deny that the sovereign advantages of co-operation are for adult human beings one of the main causes of voluntary peace.

2. In the case of apes, there is also evidence that satisfaction is found in the mere presence of others of the same species.[1] Whether this satisfaction is exclusively sexual—i.e., whether the advantage lies in the possibility of varied relations with the opposite sex—there is not sufficient evidence to determine. In so far as it is sexual, such gregariousness may easily become a source of conflict within the group. This we shall see in a moment. But in so far as pleasure is felt in the mere presence of other members of the group, there is a force binding those members together in peace.

The counterpart of the primitive sociability of the apes in children and adult human beings is obvious. Its relationship to sexual promiscuity remains as obscure in human beings as in apes, but the existence of a pleasure felt in the presence of human company could scarcely be denied. Sociability is therefore an independent cause for the existence and stability of society.[2]

3. The reasons for co-operation so far mentioned are all self-regarding advantages. They derive their importance from the existence of kinds of individual satisfaction that can only be obtained with the aid of others. We do not, however, suppose that self-regarding ends are the sole causes of peaceful co-operation. We think it obvious that in the development of the child there is to be traced the emergence of an interest in others for their own sakes, a gradual but growing recognition of the rights of others to the kinds of advantage desired by oneself; and finally in the fully developed personal relationships of friendship and love, the positive desire for the loved one's happiness as a good for oneself. From reflection and logic this care for the good of others can make the common good a personal end. The existence of a general desire for the common good is clearly a force making for peace in adult

---

[1] See Appendix.
[2] We feel it unnecessary to argue the obscure and rather formal controversy as to whether there is a specific 'herd instinct.'

society. But its power will only extend as far as the idea of the common good extends. If the common good is only felt to reach to the limits of a racial, or a geographic, or a social group, there will be no force in this recognition of the common good within the group to prevent the use of force outside and on behalf of it.

All this is very important, but it is also very obvious. It is indeed the common-place of pacifist literature. It is never difficult to find reasons for peaceful co-operation. And with such overwhelming advantages in its favour, the real problem is why peace so frequently degenerates into fighting. It is consequently much more in the study of the actual breakdown of peaceful co-operation among apes and children and grown-up people that recent descriptive work has brought new light. The work that we think to be of greatest interest falls into two parts. There is first the careful work of observation that has been carried out by Doctor Zuckermann on apes, and on children by Dr. Susan Isaacs. This does much to throw into clear perspective the most primitive causes for aggression and fighting in the absence of government. The second clue to the puzzle is to be found, in our opinion, in the mass of descriptive material laid bare by the anthropologist and in the case-papers of patients treated by the therapeutic technique of psycho-analysis. We, therefore, propose to distinguish in our brief survey between the simple causes and forms of aggressive behaviour common to apes and to human beings on the one hand and the more complicated forms exhibited by human beings alone, on the other. For an account of the complications added by the faculties of the adult human mind, we shall offer a brief and necessarily controversial interpretation of the significance of the anthropological and psycho-analytical evidence as to the origins of personal and group aggressiveness.

THE SIMPLER CAUSES OF FIGHTING

The evidence taken from the observation of the behaviour of apes and children suggests that there are three clearly separable groups of simple causes for the outbreak of fighting and the exhibition of aggressiveness by individuals.

1. One of the most common causes of fighting among

both children and apes was over the *possession* of external objects. The disputed ownership of any desired object— food, clothes, toys, females, and the affection of others—was sufficient ground for an appeal to force. On Monkey Hill disputes over females were responsible for the deaths of thirty out of thirty-three females.[1] Two points are of particular interest to notice about these fights for possession.

In the *first* place they are often carried to such an extreme that they end in the complete destruction of the objects of common desire. Toys are torn to pieces. Females are literally torn limb from limb. So over-riding is the aggression once it has begun that it not only overflows all reasonable boundaries of selfishness but utterly destroys the object for which the struggle began and even the self for whose advantage the struggle was undertaken.

In the *second* place it is observable, at least in children, that the object for whose possession aggression is started may sometimes be desired by one person only, or merely because it is desired by someone else. There were many cases observed by Dr. Isaacs where toys and other objects which had been discarded as useless were violently defended by their owners when they became the object of some other child's desire.[2] The grounds of possessiveness may, therefore, be irrational in the sense that they are derived from inconsistent judgments of value. Whether sensible or irrational, contests over possession are commonly the occasion for the most ruthless use of force among children and apes.

One of the commonest kinds of object arousing possessive desire is the notice, goodwill, affection, and service of other members of the group. Among children one of the commonest causes of quarrelling was 'jealousy'—the desire for the exclusive possession of the interest and affection of someone else, particularly the adults in charge of the children. This form of behaviour is sometimes classified as a separate cause of conflict under the name of 'rivalry' or 'jealousy.' But, in point of fact, it seems to us that it is only one variety of possessiveness. The object of desire is not a material object

---

[1] See Appendix, p. 57.
[2] This finds an interesting echo in the greater world of politics. Nations will often maintain that certain colonial territories are of no advantage to them, and yet bitterly resist any proposal to hand them over to other countries ; or rich people arguing that riches do not bless the rich, angrily resent any suggestion that they should be transferred to the poor.

—that is the only difference. The object is the interest and affection of other persons. What is wanted, however, is the exclusive right to that interest and affection—a property in emotions instead of in things. As subjective emotions and as causes of conflict, jealousy and rivalry are fundamentally similar to the desire for the uninterrupted possession of toys or food. Indeed, very often the persons, property in whom is desired, are the sources of toys and food.

Possessiveness is then in all its forms a common cause of fighting. If we are to look behind the mere facts of behaviour for an explanation of this phenomenon, a teleological cause is not far to seek. The exclusive right to objects of desire is a clear and simple advantage to the possessor of it. It carries with it the certainty and continuity of satisfaction. Where there is only one claimant to a good, frustration and the possibility of loss is reduced to a minimum. It is, therefore, obvious that, if the ends of the self are the only recognized ends, the whole powers of the agent, including the fullest use of his available force, will be used to establish and defend exclusive rights to possession.[1]

2. Another cause of aggression closely allied to possessiveness is the tendency for children and apes greatly to resent the *intrusion of a stranger* into their group. A new child in the class may be laughed at, isolated and disliked, and even set upon and pinched and bullied. A new monkey may be poked and bitten to death. It is interesting to note that it is only strangeness within a similarity of species that is resented. Monkeys do not mind being joined by a goat or a rat. Children do not object when animals are introduced to the group. Indeed, such novelties are often welcomed. But when monkeys meet a new monkey, or children a strange child, aggression often occurs. This suggests strongly that the reason for the aggression is fundamentally possessiveness. The competition of the newcomers is feared. The present members of the group feel that there will be more rivals for the food or the attention of the adults.

---

[1] This teleological rationalism does not explain the phenomenon of what we have termed irrational possessiveness. Our own explanation of the fact that a child will fight merely to possess objects because they are wanted by others is that the child in question begins to suspect that, just because someone else wants the discarded object he must have been mistaken in supposing that it was worthless. But evidence on this point is not available.

3. Finally, another common source of fighting among children is a failure or *frustration* in their own activity. A child will be prevented either by natural causes such as bad weather, or illness, or by the opposition of some adult, from doing something he wishes to do at a given moment—sail his boat or ride the bicycle. The child may also frustrate itself by failing, through lack of skill or strength, to complete successfully some desired activity. Such a child will then in the ordinary sense become ' naughty.' He will be in a bad or surly temper. And, what is of interest from our point of view, the child will indulge in aggression—attacking and fighting other children or adults. Sometimes the object of aggression will simply be the cause of frustration, a straightforward reaction. The child will kick or hit the nurse who forbids the sailing of his boat. But sometimes—indeed, frequently—the person or thing that suffers the aggression is quite irrelevant and innocent of offence. The angry child will stamp the ground or box the ears of another child when neither the ground nor the child attacked is even remotely connected with the irritation of frustration.

Of course, this kind of behaviour is so common that everyone feels it to be obvious and to constitute no serious scientific problem. That a small boy should pull his sister's hair because it is raining does not appear to the ordinary unreflecting person to be an occasion for solemn scientific enquiry. He is, as we should all say, ' in a bad temper.' Yet it is not, in fact, really obvious either why revenge should be taken on entirely innocent objects since no good to the aggressor can come of it, nor why children being miserable should seek to make others miserable also. It is just a fact of human behaviour that cannot really be deduced from any general principle of reason. But it is, as we shall see, of very great importance for our purpose. It shows how it is possible, at the simplest and most primitive level, for aggression and fighting to spring from an entirely irrelevant and partially hidden cause. Fighting to possess a desired object is straightforward and rational, however disastrous its consequences, compared with fighting that occurs because, in a different and unrelated activity, some frustration has barred the road to pleasure. The importance of this possibility for an understanding of group conflict must already be obvious.

These are the three simplest separate categories of cause we are able to observe in the evidence. One further point, however, remains to be made about the character of the fighting that occurs among apes. It is a marked characteristic of this fighting that once it has broken out anywhere it spreads with great rapidity throughout the group and draws into conflict individuals who had no part in the first quarrel and appear to have no immediate interest whatever in the outcome of the original dispute. Fighting is infectious in the highest degree. Why? It is not easy to find an answer. Whether it is that the apes who are not immediately involved feel that some advantage for themselves can be snatched from the confusion following upon the rupture of social equilibrium, or whether real advantages are involved that escape the observation of the onlooker, is not at present determined. Or it may be that the infectiousness of fighting is irrational in the same way that the irrelevant expression of aggression due to frustration is irrational. Whatever the explanation, the fact remains that fighting spreads without apparent cause or justification—that 'every dog joins a fight,' in other and older words. This excitability and the attraction which fighting may possess for its own sake is likely to be a source of great instability in any society. It is one of the most dangerous parts of our animal inheritance.

So much for the simpler forms of aggression. It is now time to consider the light thrown by anthropological and psycho-analytic evidence upon the behaviour of adult human beings.

The Further Causes of Aggressive Behaviour

So far the material from which we have sought illumination has been derived from the simple behaviour of children and apes. We must now consider more complicated behaviour. There are, as we have already pointed out, at least two relevant studies—anthropology and the case histories recorded by psycho-analysts. The present authors have most unfortunately not been able, through lack of time and assistance, to survey the vast mass of anthropological material in detail, but even such a slight study as they have been able to make suffices to show the very great importance of other causes of fighting among primitive peoples.

Before we begin this task it is necessary to make one preliminary and simple observation about the nature of adult aggression in general. It is of first importance to realise that, as far as aggressiveness and fighting is concerned, there is no noticeable improvement in the *behaviour* of adults compared with that of the most savage animals and children. If anything, it is more ruthless. The recent history of Europe establishes this conclusion with horrible insistence. There is no form of behaviour too ruthless, too brutal, too cruel for adult men and women to use against each other. Torture is becoming normal again ; the knuckle-duster and the whip, other more refined instruments of flagellation, and the armoury of mental pain are the common-place instruments of prisons and concentration camps from Japan to Spain. Men and women have been shot down without trial, soaked in petrol and burned to death, beaten to unrecognisable masses of flesh and bone, hanged by the hair and hands until they die, starved and tortured with fear and hope during the ' Reigns of Terror ' that have accompanied and succeeded the civil wars in Russia, Italy, Poland, Austria, Germany, and Spain. Cruelty knows no boundary of party or creed. It wears every kind of shirt. And over all of us there hangs, perpetual and menacing, the fear of war. No group of animals could be more aggressive or more ruthless in their aggression than the adult members of the human race.

Are there then no differences between the aggression of more primitive beings and that of adult men ? We suggest that there are only two differences. In the *first* place the aggression of adults is normally a group activity. Murder and assault are restricted to a small criminal minority. Adults kill and torture each other only when organised into political parties, or economic classes, or religious denominations, or nation states. A moral distinction is always made between the individual killing for himself and the same individual killing for some real or supposed group interest. In the *second* place, the adult powers of imagination and reason are brought to the service of the aggressive intention. Apes and children when they fight, simply fight. Men and women first construct towering systems of theology and religion, complex analyses of racial character and class structure, or moralities of group life and virility before they kill one another. Thus they fight for Protestantism or Mohammedanism, for the emancipation of the world proletariat or for the salvation of the Nordic culture, for nation or for king.   Men will die like flies for theories and exterminate each other with every instrument of destruction for abstractions.

The differences of *behaviour* are therefore not substantial. The form is the same, the results are the same. Group fighting is even more destructive than individual fighting. A machine-gun or a bomb is no less lethal because its use can be shown to be a necessity of the Class War, or noble because it brings the light of Italian civilization to the Abyssinian peoples. Now it might be argued that there is no continuity of character between the wars of civilized people and fighting of the simpler orders. We cannot, however, see any reason for supposing so. Indeed, the only question of interest appears to us to lie in the matter of causation. Are the causes exactly the same or are they changed in any important way by the greater powers and complexity of the adult human mind ?

We are therefore brought back to the question : What are the causes of aggressiveness in adult human beings ? We would maintain that anthropology and psycho-analysis suggest a number of ways in which the powers of the human mind change and add to the causes of aggression. There appear to be at least three different mechanisms discernible in the material of these two sciences.

ANIMISM

The first and most obvious of these is the cause of war revealed so very plainly by the study of primitive inter-group conflict. It consists in the universal tendency to attribute all events in the world to the deliberate activity of human or para-human *will*. All happenings, whether natural and inevitable, or human and voluntary, are attributed to the will of some being either human or anthropomorphically divine. If a thunderstorm occurs, or a hurricane visits a village, or a man is killed by a tiger, the evil is attributed either to the magic of a neighbouring tribe or the ill-will of demons and gods. In the same way, good fortune, however natural, is attributed to the deliberate intention of some other being.

This universal tendency in the human mind is termed *animism.*

It is certain that this imaginative tendency on the part of human beings leads to war. It is obvious why it should. If evil is attributed to the direct malice of neighbouring and opposing groups, the only possible protection against further evil lies in the destruction of the source of ill-will. It is, however, of great importance whether the supposed enemy is human or supernatural. If it is spiritual the natural reply will be placatory sacrifices or the harmless ritual of beating or burning or making war upon the evil spirit. The evidence discussed in the Appendix to this article shows many amusing examples of ritual warfare against the spirits undertaken by primitive peoples after some natural disaster. But if the supposed author of evil is not supernatural but human the results are neither harmless nor amusing. If the typhoon is attributed to the magic of neighbouring peoples or of dissident minorities within the tribe, then the destruction of the enemy, root and branch, is the only safe course. Hence after a thunderstorm or an accident the restless fears and hatred of the tribe will find expression in a primitive war against neighbouring tribes or the stamping out of some hapless group of victims within it. Enemies without and traitors within must be exterminated.

We think it difficult to exaggerate the frequency and importance of this cause of fighting inhuman societies of all degrees of civilization. It is a universal tendency among the simpler people of all nations to attribute evil to some person or group of persons. It is present everywhere in party politics. Every evil is loaded upon political opponents. Socialists attribute all disasters, whether economic or political, to ' capitalists ' or ' the capitalist class.' Conservatives think it obvious that the last uncontrollable and world-wide depression in trade was due to the ' bad government ' of the Socialists in this country. Other movements find different and more peculiar scapegoats in ' the bankers,' or ' the Jews,' or ' the Russians.' In each case what is noticeable and dangerous is that a vast power and a deep malignity is attributed to the inimical group. The supposed malignity is often purely illusory. The attributed power transcends all reality. When the open conflict of party politics is suppressed by an authoritarian regime the tendency is exaggerated rather than reduced. Some unfortunate minority within the group—' the Jews ' or ' the Kulaks '—become the source of all evil, the scapegoat of all disaster. Or an overwhelming hatred is conceived for another nation. Out of these real terrors and derivative hatreds merciless persecutions and international wars are likely to spring.

We shall go on to show that the sources of aggression among human beings are much more complicated than either the simple causes operating in animals or this common habit of attributing everything to some human agency. Yet it should be obvious that much of the behaviour of large groups can be explained by the categories of cause we have already discussed. Possessiveness, frustration, animism are potent causes of conflict between groups—whether parties, classes or states. After we have discussed the complex history of aggression within the individual we shall have reason to revert to these simpler forms of behaviour. It seems probable that the complex character of the civilized individual undergoes a degeneration or simplification into simpler forms and simpler reactions when he is caught up into and expresses himself through the unity of the group. The behaviour of the group is in an important sense simpler and more direct than the behaviour of the individual. But in the meantime we must consider the light thrown by psycho-analysis upon the history and development of aggressive impulses in the civilized adult.

The Transformation of Aggressive Impulses— Displacement and Projection

What light does psycho-analytic evidence throw upon the problem of adult aggression ? It is, of course, impossible to consider at all adequately the mass of material and theory comprised in the work of this school of psychology. Part of it is summarized in the Appendix. All that we can attempt at this point is a brief account of the main conclusions—as they appear to us—of the evidence. It is scarcely necessary to point out that our views are only one interpretation of the data, and although we think our interpretation to be the most accurate, it could only be verified by the kind of practical test that we suggest at the end of this article.

We suggest tentatively therefore that the evidence of psycho-analysis justifies the following conclusions :

1. That the *primary* causes of aggression (and of peaceful co-operation) are identical with those of children and apes. The character of the *id*—or complex of instinctive impulses—does not change materially as the individual grows older. The same sources of satisfaction—food, warmth, love, society—are desired and the same sources of conflict—desire for exclusive possession of the sources of satisfaction, or aggression arising from a sense of frustration—are present. But in the life of most children there is a controlling or warping influence present in a varying degree, that of *authority*. The child is denied for various reasons—good or bad—an open and uninterrupted access to the means of its satisfaction. It is denied the breast or bottle, the toy or the company of adults at the time or to the extent that it wishes. The evidence seems overwhelming that such frustration leads to a violent reaction of fear, hatred, and aggression. The child cries or screams or bites or kicks. We are not for the moment concerned with the question whether this frustration is desirable or not. We are simply concerned with its results. The result is ' bad temper ' or ' naughtiness '—a resentment of frustration. This original resentment and the aggression to which it leads we would call *simple aggression*.

Further development turns in our view, upon the way in which this simple aggression is treated. The statistically normal method of treatment is, we suggest, further frustration or *punishment*. The child is slapped or beaten or subjected to moral instruction—taught that its behaviour is wrong or wicked. Again we are not concerned with the question of the rightness or wrongness of this procedure, but only with its consequences. We suggest that the result of punishment is to present the child with a radical conflict—either he must control the expression of his simple aggression or suffer the punishment and the loss of love that simple aggression in a regime of discipline necessarily entails.

This conflict in the child is in our view an important source of aggressiveness in the adult. The conflict itself is a conflict between a fundamental tendency to resent frustration and the fear of punishment or, what is just as important, the fear of the loss of love. To the child the parent[1] is both the source of satisfactions and the source of frustration. To express aggression is to endanger the life of the goose that lays the golden eggs. Not to express simple aggression towards original objects is the task that faces the child. Now one result of the child's attempt to resolve the conflict is called *repression*.[2] Much has been written about the nature and consequences of repression. The hypothesis of the existence and independent functioning of an unconscious mind has been elaborated to explain the analytical evidence, and a whole literature of theory has been built upon this idea. We are not here primarily concerned with psycho-analytic theory and we feel that the main contributions of the evidence to an understanding of the sources of aggressiveness can be explained quite simply. The overwhelming fact established by the evidence is that aggression, however deeply hidden or disguised, does not disappear. It appears later and in other forms. It is not destroyed. It is safe to conclude from the evidence that it cannot be destroyed. Whether we conceive simple aggression stimulated by frustration as a quantity of energy that has to be released somewhere, or whether we imagine that a secret and unconscious character is formed that is aggressive although the superficial character is peaceful, or whether we simply suppose that a certain kind of character is formed, peaceful in certain directions and aggressive in others—is a matter of comparative indifference and mainly of terminology. The fundamental fact is that the punishment of simple aggression results in the appearance of aggression in other forms. The boy, instead of striking his father whom he fears, strikes a smaller boy whom he does not fear. Disguised aggression has made the boy into a bully. The girl who dares not scream at her mother grows up to hate other women. Again a character has been formed by a simple aggressiveness that has been controlled but not destroyed. And in the same way revolutionaries who hate ordered government, nationalists who hate foreign peoples, individuals who hate bankers, Jews, or their political opponents, may be exhibiting characteristics

[1] Throughout this article we use the term ' parent ' to refer to the person or persons, whoever it may be, who are responsible for looking after the child—whether they are in fact parents or nurses or aunts or teachers.
[2] The tendency to aggression is not the only thing that may be repressed. Certain other impulses that are punished or condemned by adults or repudiated by the child himself may also be repressed. Much psycho-analytic evidence and theory is concerned with the repression of these other impulses—particularly the sexual impulses.

that have been formed by the suppression of simple aggression in their childhood education.[1] These aggressive aspects of adult character and the aggressiveness to which they lead we call *transformed aggression*. It is the displaced and unrecognized fruit of suppressed simple aggression.

2. The second great contribution of psycho-analytic evidence is to show the kind of transformations that simple aggression undergoes as the adult faculties develop. The fundamental problem of the child, is, as we have seen, a double one : that of self-control and of *ambivalence*. In order to escape punishment the child must prevent its aggressive impulses from appearing—it must control its natural aggression. But this is not the whole of the problem. The parent has become for the child the object of two incompatible emotions—love and hatred. As a source of satisfaction and companionship the parent is greatly beloved. As a source of frustration and punishment the parent is greatly feared and hated. The evidence demonstrates overwhelmingly that such a double attitude to one person puts a terrible emotional strain upon the child. In the growth and development of character a number of imaginative and intellectual efforts are made to alleviate or avoid the severity of this internal conflict.

One other aspect of the subjective life must be mentioned before we examine the processes by which internal strain or anxiety is reduced to a minimum—and that is the question of *moral judgment*. We are not at this juncture concerned with the theories of the origin of what the moralist calls the conscience and the psycho-analyst the *super-ego*. It is obvious that persons are deeply influenced in their behaviour and their feeling by what they think they ought to do and ought to be— their ' sense of duty.' We think it also clear from the evidence of psycho-analysis that the content of this moral sense—the total of the things a man feels to be his duty—is made up partly of objective moral judgments and partly of compulsions arising from the teaching and discipline of childhood.[2] The

---

[1] We are not for a moment suggesting either (*a*) that logical and objective cases cannot be argued in favour of revolutions, wars, and persecutions, or (*b*) that the positive valuation of such things as justice, liberty, and other social values may not reasonably involve a hatred of their opposites. We are only suggesting that the repression of simple aggression may result in these forms of hatred. The objective cases of these schools of thought are in every case different in kind from the personal and subjective elements in their supporters' view of them.

[2] And partly of the remnants of the exaggerated and fantastic moral judgments of the child.

moral sense is neither wholly rational nor wholly subjective and irrational. It is partly the one and partly the other. But whatever the origin of the moral sense, there is conclusive evidence that it can become the source of immense burdens of shame and guilt, both to the child and to the adult. Again we think that the available evidence demonstrates beyond question that such guilt in the adult is composed partly of a sensible consciousness of moral failure, partly of an irrational fear of punishment derived from the experiences and wild imagination of childhood and partly of an half-conscious recognition of the dangerous aggressive impulses within himself. All these elements combine to make a considerable burden of guilt—acknowledged or unacknowledged—for most individuals, a burden that rises to intolerable levels for depressed and suicidal subjects.

There is, then, much support in the empirical work of character psychology for the theological doctrine of a 'man divided against himself.' Not only do we both love and hate the same people, but we are divided into an impulsive and appetitive character, only part of which we acknowledge, on the one hand, and a stern and inescapable sense of duty which is often partially unrecognized, on the other.' These divisions of our being are at war with each other and are responsible for much of the unhappiness of individual life and are the direct source of the universal phenomenon of *morbid anxiety*.

It is to reduce anxiety and guilt to a minimum and to resolve the conflict of ambivalence that the major psychological mechanisms are developed. These are of two kinds—*displacement* and *projection* : both of them are frequently used for the expression of transformed aggression.

1. *Displacement.* This is perhaps the simplest mechanism of all. Several examples of it have already been cited. It is extremely common in political and social affairs. It consists in the transference of fear or hatred or love from the true historical object to a secondary object. The secondary object may be loved or hated for its own sake, but to the sensible degree of feeling is added an intensity derived from the transference to it of irrelevant passion. The child is thwarted by its father and then bullies a smaller child. The father is reprimanded by his employer of whom he is afraid and then is angry with his son. A girl both loves and feels jealous of

her mother. To deal with this situation she may direct her loving feelings towards her school-mistress and feel free to hate her mother more completely. A boy may hate his father through familial discipline and grow up to hate all authority and government. He would be a revolutionary under any regime. Children who both love and hate their parents grow up to love their own country blindly and uncritically and to hate foreign countries with equal blindness and unreason. They have succeeded in displacing their opposite emotions to different objects.

The tendency to identify the self with the community is so common as to be obvious.[1] The transference of the predominant feelings of childhood from parents to the organs of political life—to the State and the parties in it—is almost universal. Hence the importance of symbolical figureheads and governors, Kings and Führers. Hence the fanaticism and violence of political life. Hence the comparative weakness of reason and moderation in political affairs.

The advantage to the individual of these displacements or transferences of emotion from their historically relevant objects should be obvious. In the *first* place the confusion and strain of the ambivalent relation is often resolved. Instead of both loving and hating the mother it is possible to love the school-mistress and to hate more freely—however secretly—the person who was originally both loved and hated with equal intensity. Instead of both loving and hating the same adults it is possible to love the nation or the Communist Party with pure devotion and hate the Germans or the ' Capitalist Class ' with frenzy. In either case the world of emotional objects is redeemed from its original chaos—simplicity and order are restored to it. Action and purposive life is possible again.[2] In the *second* place the displacement is often, indeed usually, towards a safer object. It is safer to kick a smaller boy than to kick

---

[1] Nor is such an identification by any means wholly unreasonable. After all, the communities in which we are brought up have entered into us and made us what we are. It is natural that we should feel that what happens to them happens also to us more personally than they really do.

[2] When a suitable division of emotion and transference is carried out suddenly the phenomenon of ' conversion ' often appears. Persons suddenly decide to give all their devotion to the Church or Party, and all their hatred to the ' world ' or the Party's enemies. Conflicts suddenly disappear and a frustrated and unhappy individual becomes a confident and happy Christian or Communist or National Socialist. Of course, which of these things he becomes is determined by other forces—including the social and historical environment.

one's father. It is safer for the individual to hate the capitalists than to hate his wife, or to hate the Russians than to hate his employers. Thus fear and anxiety—though not banished— is reduced. Happiness is increased. Of course greater safety is not always reached in any objective sense. To join the Communist Party instead of divorcing one's wife may result in imprisonment and even death. To become a patriot may mean early enlistment and a premature grave, when the alternative was objectively less dangerous. But unless we are to deny the teleological interpretation of human affairs altogether it seems obvious that the internal conflicts of fear and guilt are alleviated by displacement. And there is ample direct evidence to support this view.[1]

From our present point of view the importance of this mechanism can scarcely be exaggerated. Adult aggression, as we have seen, is normally carried out in group activity. Political parties make civil war. Churches make religious war. States make international war. These various kinds of groups can attract absolute loyalty and canalize torrents of hatred and murder—through the mechanism of displacement. Individuals can throw themselves into the life and work of groups because they find a solution to their own conflicts in them. The stores of explosive violence in the human atom are released by and expressed in group organization. The power of the group for aggression is derived partly from the sensible and objective judgments of men, but chiefly in our view, by their power to attract to themselves the displaced hatred and destructiveness of their members. Displacement, though not the ultimate cause, is a direct channel of the ultimate causes of war.

2. *Projection.* A second group of mechanisms that are of the greatest importance in understanding individual and social behaviour are those of projection. It is not so simple a mechanism as that of displacement, but the psycho-analytic evidence demonstrates that it is of frequent occurrence in social life. The mechanism consists in imagining that other

---

[1] It is also important to realize that the displacement may be temporary. Certain displacements of hatred or love involve further conflict and guilt. Thus the boy who transfers his hatred to his father into bullying may feel after a time, extremely guilty about his cruelty. Members of extreme parties may find themselves involved in blood guilt. Thus displacement, always bringing temporary relief, may lead in vicious circles more and more deeply into conflict towards final breakdown or suicide.

individuals are really like our own unrecognized and un-
accepted selves. It is the projection of our own characters
upon others.

There are two parts of subjective character that the individual
' projects upon ' others in this way—two kinds of unrecognized
motives of his own that he imagines are animating other
people : first his real but unrecognized impulses, and secondly
his unrecognized conscience. In the first case we suppose others
to be wicked in the ways that we do not admit ourselves to
be wicked ; in the second we suppose them to be censorious
and restrictive in ways that we do not recognize our own
super-ego to criticize and restrain us.

(a) *The Projection of Impulse.* Examples of the way in which
people project upon others the evil that is really in themselves
are not far to seek. There are men and women who imagine
that everyone's hand is against them ; persons who are mean
and parsimonious and who assume that everyone else is seeking
to swindle them. Persecution manias or *paranoia* contain, as
well as simple animism, an element of this mechanism. In
all these cases it seems obvious to us that the individual is either
assuming that people will treat him as he wishes to treat them,
or that he imagines them to be animated by the motives and
impulses that are really his own. The miser attributes to others
his own impulse to swindle. The paranoid imagines the
object of his fears to be animated by his own wicked and
destructive passions.

To the authors, most cases of political persecution seem to
be of this kind. We have already seen that much of this
behaviour can be explained in terms of the simplest animism
—the tendency to blame some human will for all disasters.
But the existence of such a tendency does not explain why
persecution continues when no disaster is present or threatening.
And yet they do continue after all reasonable and unreasonable
occasion has passed. Almost all authoritarian regimes treasure
a pet object of persecution indefinitely. The National Socialists
persecute the Communists and the Jews ; the Bolsheviks
persecute the Trotskyist and the Kulaks. It is commonly said
that regimes ' need a scapegoat.' We suggest that over and
above any objective reasons for persecution—the need for an
excuse in case of failure or the desire to crush opposition by
fear—and explaining the continuation of persecution long after

the objective reasons have lost their force, there is an element of pure projection. The persecuted minorities are made to carry the projected wickedness of the dominant masses. They are truly the scapegoat of the people, not only in the sense that they are hated and despised, but also that they are made literally to bear the ' sins of the people.' We think it important to realize that the National Socialists seriously believe that the Jews are responsible for national degradation—that the Communists seriously believe that the Kulaks threatened the regime—and they believe these things against all evidence because they have successfully projected upon these groups so much of the disruptive elements within themselves. The hated minorities are genuinely thought to be the cause of disruption because they have become the external symbol of internal wickedness.

The advantage of this mechanism is again obvious. It reduces anxiety to force the enemy outside the gate of one's soul. It is better to hate other people for meanness and to bear the fear of their ill-will than to hate oneself for being miserly. To see wickedness in others, though terrifying, is better than to be divided against oneself. It avoids the terrible burden of guilt.

Its importance for the understanding of group aggressiveness is also plain. If it is possible to project upon other groups all the evil within the group, then, as in the case of simple animism, the forces of hatred and fear against the external group will grow more and more intense. If Communists can persuade themselves that all aggressiveness and cruelty is with the Fascists, and Fascists that all treachery and destructiveness is with the Communists, then civil war can be fought with better will and greater ferocity on both sides. If Englishmen owning a quarter of the world can feel that all ruthless imperialism is exhibited by Germany, and Germany with the most powerful army in Europe can feel herself threatened by Russia, then the selfishness of the one group and the aggressiveness of the other can be justified without being reduced. Projection is an admirable mechanism for turning the other man into the aggressor, for making hatred appear as a passion for righteousness, for purifying the hate-tormented soul. By this means all war is made into religious war—a crusade for truth and virtue.

(b) *The Projection of Conscience.* Finally, to complete the story, there is the projection of the conscience. In order to escape the pains of self-condemnation, the individual projects upon others the moral judgments and condemnation of his own heart. This leads to a particular form of paranoia or persecution mania—in which persons resent, not only the real, but also purely imaginary moral judgments and legal restraints imposed by the State. It is particularly common among the revolutionary opponents of an existing order. Communists exaggerate enormously the degree and deliberateness of capitalist repression. National Socialists in opposition exaggerated absurdly the oppressions of *das System.* Both parties, all the while, intending to create a far more repressive system themselves. This projection of internal moral censorship, while of great interest in explaining many of the phenomena of political life, is not of central importance in understanding the causes of international war. Displacement and the projection of impulse are the great channels of transformed aggression. The projection of the super-ego is chiefly a cause of revolution and civil war.[1]

We have now completed our survey of the causes of aggression in human beings. We have suggested that there is no substantial difference in behaviour, that adults are just as cruel—or more so—just as aggressive, just as destructive as any group of animals or monkeys. The only difference in our view is one of psychological and intellectual mechanism. The causes of simple aggression—possessiveness, strangeness, frustration—are common to adults and simpler creatures. But a repressive discipline drives the simple aggression underground—to speak in metaphors—and it appears in disguised forms. These transformations are chiefly those of displacement and projection. These mechanisms have as their immediate motive the reduction of anxiety and the resolution of the conflicts of ambivalence and guilt. They result in the typical form of adult aggressiveness—aggressive personal relations of all kinds—but above all in group aggression : party conflict,

---

[1] The projection of the super-ego is a reason for hating and attacking any form of government. If, therefore, the League of Nations or any collective security system became strong there would then arise, if our theory be true, aggressive revolutionary minorities within the collective system. This is an important point made by Dr. Glover. We shall discuss its political significance in the later sections of this part of the article.

civil war, wars of religion, and international war. The group life gives sanction to personal aggressiveness. The mobilization of transformed aggression gives destructive power to groups. Aggression takes on its social form. And to justify it—to explain the group aggression to the outside world and to the group itself in terms that make it morally acceptable to the members of the group—great structures of intellectual reasoning— theories of history and religion and race—are built up. The impulses are rationalized. The hatred is justified. And it is typical of the complexity of human affairs that something in these theories is always true. But most is false, most of it a mere justification of hatred, a sickening and hypocritical defence of cruelty. This is particularly true of the political persecutions of dictatorships. We must now try to apply the conclusions of this evidence to the theory of the causes of war.

THE THEORY OF WAR

We hold that the evidence summarized above suggests a certain theory of the causes of war. In the absence of government—the organization of force to preserve the peace—we hold that a group of monkeys or children or men can only achieve at the best, an unstable social equilibrium. It may very well be that an appreciation of the advantages of co-operation and an agreement to continue it will preserve the peace for some time. But underneath there is a powerful and 'natural' tendency to resort to force in order to secure the possession of desired objects, or to overcome a sense of frustration, or to resist the encroachment of strangers, or to attack a scapegoat. Fighting and peaceful co-operation are equally 'natural' forms of behaviour, equally fundamental tendencies in human relations. Peaceful co-operation predominates—there is much more peace than war—but the willingness to fight is so widely distributed in space and time that it must be regarded as a basic pattern of human behaviour. The cause of the transition from one to the other is simply when some change in the circumstances of the group alters the balance between the desire for co-operation and the conflicting desire to obtain self-regarding ends by force. New females are introduced into the community of monkeys, food runs short, rain falls, or a new toy is given to a group of children. The pre-existing balance of desires is disturbed. The advantages to be gained by aggression grow greater. Fighting begins and spreads throughout the group. Social equilibrium is destroyed. Of course we are not arguing that any real advantage is secured by the appeal to force. In the vast majority of cases the parties to a struggle would all be better off had they been able to continue co-operating with each other. All that we wish to insist upon is the universality of the tendency not to think so and the consequent willingness of minorities to fight.

What differences are made to the operation of these primitive forces by the development of more complex societies and cultures ? For the moment we are not concerned with the prevention of aggression. To this vital matter we shall return. We are only concerned with the form of its expression. What activities of a developed society influence the form aggression takes ? We suggest that there are two such activities—that of education and that of government.

1. The character of parental and familial control we have already discussed. In so far as the emotional education of the child throughout human society involves apetitive frustration, and in so far as intellectual education develops powers of reasoning and imagination, the forms of aggression change. It is rationalized, explained, and justified. It is displaced and projected. Above all, it is expressed in the life and activities of groups. Religious, economic, and political groups—churches, classes, and parties—release for the individual the aggression he dare not express for himself. And the greatest of all these groups—at least in the modern world—is the State. It is by an identification of the self with the State and by the expression of aggression through it, that the individual has in recent times chiefly exhibited his aggressive impulses. Not exclusively so, for religious war and civil war have played an important part, but the great wars and the great loss of life have been in wars between nation states.

2. It is natural that it should be so because the nation State normally succeeds in preventing or controlling all other forms of aggression. The existence of government—with its apparatus of force—enormously increases the penalties of private aggression. Not only does the rationalizing mind and

the conscience of mankind condemn private fighting and killing, but the social will to co-operation creates an instrument of force to control and punish any criminal minority that disturbs the peace. Hence private aggression is not only condemned by the conscience—it is also punished by the law. And so long as the State maintains supreme power, the same thing is true of all kinds of group aggression other than its own. Political and racial parties are prevented from taking the law into their own hands. Tendencies to civil war are successfully repressed.[1] In such circumstances it is natural, in our view, that transformed aggression should be chiefly canalized by, and flow unimpeded through, the State organizations of common endeavour and military adventure. In the service of the State the rationalized and transferred impulses of men find their last remaining and freest outlet.

What then causes the State to embark on war? We offer two conclusions in answer to this question. In the *first* place, as we have already mentioned, the expression of aggression on a group scale appears to restore to it simplicity and directness. In the civilized adult the original and simple causes for fighting are forgotten and overlaid with every kind of excuse and transformation. But when aggression is made respectable by manifestation through the corporate will of the group it resumes much of its amoral simplicity of purpose. Indeed, positive moral obligation becomes attached to it. Nations will fight for simple possession, or through hatred due to animism, or because of national frustration, in a direct and shameless way that would be quite impossible for their individual members. The mutual approval of the members of the group makes conscienceless aggression possible. Hence states will fight for the same reasons as children fight. But not only for those things. In the *second* place states may fight, in our submission, because of the pressure of transformed aggression within their members. The members of the State may be so educated, so frustrated, and so unhappy, that the burden of internal aggression may become intolerable. Such

---

[1] Of course, the State does not always succeed in preventing group aggression within itself from breaking out. Not only is there occasional rioting, but in recent years democratic Governments, have frequently allowed Party groups to grow up and make revolutions and civil war. Civil war or group aggression within the State means the breakdown of internal sovereignty.

peoples—or the dominant groups within them[1]—may constitute in a real sense aggressive nations. They have reached a point at which war has become a psychological necessity. Ambivalence is so severe, internal conflict so painful, fear and hatred of the scapegoat so intense, that a resolution of the crisis can only be found in war. In such cases war will be fought without adequate objective cause. It will have an objective occasion, some trifling incident or dispute, but the real effective causes will be elsewhere, within the tormented souls of the members of the aggressor nation. Such national neuroses can exhibit any or all of the general psychological mechanisms that we have already examined—animism, displacement, the projection of impulse, or the projection of conscience. Thus nations will exhibit the aggressiveness typical of apes and also the much more complex and obscure aggressiveness typical of humanity. They will fight because they are disciplined, because they are divided against themselves, because they have constructed mythical enemies and conjured terrors out of the darkness, because they are paranoid or sadistic. The balance of impulse between co-operation and force has been shifted against the advantages of peace.

This then is our theory of international war. War occurs because fighting is a fundamental tendency in human things —a form of behaviour called forth by certain simple situations in animals, children, human groups, and whole nations. It is a fundamentally pluralistic theory of international war. If the theory is true, then it follows that nations *can* fight only because they are able to release the explosive stores of transformed aggression, but they *do* fight for any of a large number of reasons. They may fight because of simple acquisitiveness, or simple frustration, or a simple fear of strangers. They may fight because of displaced hatred, or projected hates or fears. There is no single all-embracing cause—no single villain of the piece, no institution nor idea that is wholly to blame. In

---

[1] We should mention in this context that we are quite aware that there is much more to be said on this subject than we have space to say or the learning to write. Large nations are not simple homogeneous groups. Power in them is divided between many groups and dispersed over a varying proportion of the members of the nation. The analysis of the group structure within the nation and of the distribution of power among the sub-groups is a task for sociology and sociologists. We are not competent to perform it. We are only concerned with the type of impulse dominating groups with power, whether those groups are the whole or only part of the nation.

this sense the theory stands in marked contrast to almost all accepted theories of the day. To two of these we shall turn in a moment, but before we do so there are one or two further comments to be made in explanation of the theory here defended.

In the *first* place it should be obvious to the reader that in one sense the theory is nothing more than enlightened common sense. It is no overwhelming novelty to show that war is a common form of human behaviour. It resembles the familiar doctrine that ' to fight is only human nature.' The authors wish to emphasize this. They wish to make no claims to great originality. The value of the evidence here gathered together is simply that it shows the grounds upon which, and the form in which, such a common-sense theory can be held. It seeks to describe in greater detail the kinds of situation that call forth the impulses to aggression. It traces the causes of simple aggression in individuals, and follows it through the disguised forms it exhibits in them, into its social manifestations. It shows how and why war is a chronic disease of the social organism. It fills out a simple theory with detail and reason. It throws doubt upon all other theories. That is all.

In the *second* place, it will be as well to say something of the other reasons given by human beings for a willingness to fight in aggressive wars.[1] They fall into two groups. There are first the reasons given by those who defend war as a political institution. It is claimed by such people that war permits and demands the display in a marked degree of certain fundamental human virtues—virility, courage, loyalty, a care for the common good. It has further been suggested to us that this fact, or the belief that this is a fact, is one of the common reasons why individuals are prepared to fight. Now it is obvious that the bare statement that war gives an opportunity for the display of certain personal virtues is true. Moreover, the statement is plainly a most important part of the stock-in-trade of militarist propaganda. But that does not carry us far in assessing the effectiveness of this argument in making people willing to fight. It is a commonplace of moral teaching throughout the history of civilization that these virtues can

---

[1] We are distinguishing here between aggressive wars and police ' wars '—or the use of force to protect peace and ensure law. See Part III.

be displayed equally well in peaceful competition and peaceful co-operation. It is a platitude to point out that courage, loyalty, and virility are required as much by the arts of peace as by the arts of war. Pioneer navigation on the sea or in the air, dangerous occupations of social value demand courage and comradeship of the highest order. The problem is not why the virtues of strength attract and compel human endeavour, but why the exercise of these virtues in the work of destruction and death make so wide an appeal. The appeal of adventure is intelligible, but why the appeal of killing? We suggest that while the desire for a life of strength and virtue is no doubt a subsidiary cause of the willingness to fight, it is impossible to deny that the peculiar sensitiveness of people to the propaganda of war must be attributed to the existence of an underlying willingness to kill. No other explanation seems to us to account for the ease with which courage and virility can be associated with war.

Then similarly it has been suggested to us that the mere desire for change and movement on the part of most individuals is an independent cause of a willingness to fight. Most people, it is suggested, are discontented with their lot in greater or less degree. They are conscious of frustration, disappointment, and even despair. A war is an opportunity to start again, to see new things and to escape from old chains. There is no question that there is a great deal in this—that many persons are released by war from situations in which they are bored or unhappy. They have, in that sense, a reasonable motive for welcoming war. But is that all that there is to be said? We hardly think so. Does anyone suppose that any kind of general disturbance would be equally welcome? An earthquake that struck half England would stir up enough excitement to release and change the lives of most of its inhabitants. Does anyone really suppose that such a disaster would awaken the passions of exaltation and enthusiasm that are so frequently evoked by war. It seems to us absurd to suppose so. It is not the fact of a general disturbance that excites men, but the kind of disturbance in which hatred and destruction may run and be glorified. It is not the excitement of change, but the excitement of blood that fills the streets with cheering crowds and sends the first—though not the last—regiments into war with trumpets. People are less sensible and more savage than these rational theories of the willingness to fight seems to suppose.

But in the third place, let us at once make clear, that there is nothing in the least alarmist or defeatist in the theory here advanced. We do not hold, nor think it possible to hold, that because war is a chronic social disease it is necessarily an incurable disease. Not only have we emphasized throughout this article that the forces making for peaceful co-operation have been more powerful in history than the forces making for war, but we have not yet considered the implications of our evidence for the theory of the *cure* of war—the therapeutic as distinct from the causal problem. This we shall attempt to do after we have examined the bearing of this theory upon other theories of the cause of war. All that it is necessary to do at this stage is to repeat and emphasize these three points :

1. Far more of the time and vitality of any nation has been absorbed in past history by the activities of peaceful co-operation than by war. The impulses to peace are therefore more powerful than the impulses to war. Hence the problem —how can they be further strengthened ?

2. The governments of states have been successful in preserving comparative peace within their countries for centuries at a time. Is it not possible then, that the expression of aggression can be permanently prevented or controlled by government ?

3. We have only argued that the social and educational environments of the past have in fact produced certain ' quantities ' of aggression. Is it possible that different societies and different educations might produce less ?

II

What is the bearing of the theory here outlined upon other and more popular theories of the cause of war ? It is, as we have seen, itself a simple theory. But it has important consequences for the other theories of war commonly held to-day. We wish to bring out the implications of what we have said for two of the most prevalent contemporary theories—the theory that ' war is due to capitalism,' and the theory that ' war is due to nationalism.'

THE ECONOMIC CAUSES OF WAR

In its simplest form it is almost inconceivable that the theory that 'war is due to capitalism' should be true. Capitalism as an historical type of system—its distinctive characteristics of unlimited acquisitiveness, rationalism in technique, and rapid expansion—is not more than three hundred years old. War as a social habit is far older than that. It is therefore difficult to see how the one could have caused the other. Of course it is *conceivable* that by pure accident the fundamental causes of war suffered a violent and complete change in character just when capitalism began. It is not inconceivable that at the beginning of the seventeenth century the purpose and cause of war underwent a complete change—that up to 1600 war had been due to one set of causes, and that after that date the causes became entirely different. It is conceivable, but it is in the highest possible degree improbable. War is a continuously recurring phenomenon throughout recorded history. There is almost no period in which war is not taking place somewhere in the world. It occurs among primitive peoples, in the ancient world, in the ' dark ages,' in the medieval world, and in modern times. It occurs in almost every civilization girdling the world from the Far East, through Europe and Africa to the remote civilizations of Peru.[1] It seems more than improbable that with the beginning of capitalism in Western Europe the causes of war became utterly changed. Yet, unless this happened, it cannot be true in any complete sense that capitalism is the cause of war. An effect cannot precede its cause. Capitalism cannot be the cause of war if the same kind of war occurred before capitalism began.

The same type of theory can, however, be put in more persuasive forms. It may, instead, be contended that war is always due to *class conflict*, or that war is always due to *economic causes*. These phenomena are, unlike capitalism, co-extensive in time with war. Throughout recorded history

---

[1] It has been shown by Prof. Ginsberg that only thirteen out of three hundred and eleven groups of primitive peoples did not frequently fight, and most of this small number did not meet each other much. The only civilization which may not have been warlike—quoted by pacifists—is that of the Indus. All others make use of war.

societies have exhibited an hierarchical structure and the consequent division of society into class groups.[1] Between these groups conflict is at least possible. In the same way economic activities, the struggle for wealth and conflicts over the division of the social product, are as ancient as society itself. It is therefore possible that war is the consequence of these phenomena and we must examine the bearing of our theory upon the contention that it is. It should at once be obvious that there is no complete contradiction between the second of these views and the theory we advocate. From our point of view the theory that war is due to economic causes—to the struggle for wealth—is not wrong but merely incomplete. We have emphasized ourselves that one of the commonest causes of fighting at the primitive and pre-adult levels is over the right to the uninterrupted enjoyment, or property in, sources of advantage or imagined advantage. Consequently it is perfectly compatible with our theory, indeed implied by it, that wars are frequently fought by groups and by nations to gain possession of territories, markets, or other groups of persons. The shameless and ruthless acquisitiveness of nations merely represents to us the emergence at the group level, of primitive individual behaviour, strengthened and justified by group approval. Economic occasions for war resulting from the a-moral acquisitiveness of groups, we should expect on our theory to be frequent in history, as indeed they are.

The false element in the theory would lie in any suggestion that economic causes are the *sole* cause of war. Holding a pluralist theory about the causes of fighting, we wish to question the doctrine that the acquisitiveness of nations or of groups within the nation is the sole cause of war. The desire to possess sources of advantage is not the only cause of international war. Even at the simplest level of human behaviour the frustration of other ends is shown by the evidence to be a different and separable cause of fighting, while at a higher level the habits of animistic thought, displacement and projection can become the cause of national aggressiveness. Thus it comes about that nations may go to war for other than economic causes. They may, for example, be willing to go to war because

---

[1] The ' class ' structure in a primitive tribe may be extremely simple, and may not be associated with economic privilege. The only superior group may be a meeting of the ' elders '—the older men. They may constitute a power group or political class.

a harsh and restrictive form of education and discipline is common within the nation, or because an economic depression has increased the feeling of frustration and self-hatred in individual life. For these and many other reasons, quite unconnected with rational or irrational acquisitiveness, war-like regimes may come to power or group aggression take place.

One of the most obvious types of these group frustrations is the loss of a war against another people. Defeat will generate hatred and lead to internal civil strife or renewed external aggression, either against the nations responsible for the defeat, or against someone else. Hence the frequency of serial wars and prolonged rivalries between tribes and nations. Of these the tragic and enduring animosities of Europe are a terrible example.

Hence there seems to us no sense in which war is necessarily and always due to economic causes. What, then, is to be made of the other alternative—that it is always due to class conflict—that war between nations is always the by-product of the struggle between classes for mastery within the nation? It is not always clear how exactly it is supposed that the internal struggle precipitates the external war, but presumably the two things may be connected in either or both of the following ways. Either it may be supposed that the passions and hatred engendered in the Class War can easily be deflected into national war—that the Class War stokes up the fires of aggression and the tension thus generated can explode in any direction ; or it may be suggested that every international war is a move in the strategy of the Class War—that the exploiting class of one nation uses the instruments of propaganda to arouse the fears and hatred of the exploited class and, having called them up, directs them against an external group.

Now there is obviously a great deal of truth in these doctrines. Just as severe internal familial conflict or repression is likely to make a person aggressive, so will internal class conflict and repression be likely to make a nation aggressive. It is not quite so obvious how the process of deflection is brought about. How can hatred that is already rationalized into class loyalty be deflected into that of national patriotism? It is not, however, inconceivable that this could be done, and it is a

familiar fact that nations in which class conflict is particularly
sharp are often war-like—though this is by no means always
the case. But the working of the second mechanism—in which
external war is used as one move in the strategy of internal
conflict—is obvious and not infrequent. Wars have often been
fought that were in the interests of the governing group or
class within a community and were not in the interests of the
great mass of the community. A dictatorship faced by the
threat of internal revolution may be able to use the apparatus
of propaganda and coercion in its hands to inflame and force
a people into war. A ring of armament manufacturers may
finance war-like propaganda or use their influence to push
foreign policy in the direction of war. All these things are
possible and historical examples of them exist.

Yet in our view the theory that class conflict must lead
to war or that international war is the by-product of class war
seems to us incomplete and inaccurate. In the *first* place there
is the question of exclusiveness. Many wars are not fought
because the Government is in danger. Very strong governments make war. Many nations in which the internal group
conflict is very severe are peaceful in their relations with
external peoples.[1] Fighting in all ways similar to war occurs,
it is scarcely necessary to repeat, among individuals, children,
and apes. In such groups there is no class structure and
therefore no class war. The connection between class conflict
and war can in no possible way exhaust the causes of war. But
secondly, the ' class war ' theory depends upon the implicit
but vital assumption that some force—' propaganda ' or ' the
Press ' or the ' capitalist class '—can inflame the people and
make them mad. It is, of course, perfectly reasonable to contend that a strong dictatorial regime can drive an *unwilling*
people into war. But in order to explain the fact that democratic nations, whose governments depend upon popular
suffrage and are sensitive to public opinion, often wage war,
and shamelessly aggressive wars at that, the advocates of the
' class war ' theory of international war are forced back upon
the view that some interested minority manipulates the organs
of propaganda in order to madden and frighten the people
into a willingness to fight. It is precisely this underlying
assumption of their theory that pure economic or class war

[1] We think Spain to be an obvious example in this category.

theorists fail to explain. Why is it that people can be roused
in this way? Even if it were true that in a capitalist system
all the methods of propaganda could be mobilized by one
sectional group, how is it that the national passions can so
easily be roused to fighting? We do not imagine that even
the most orthodox exponents of the views we are discussing
would wish to deny that war is often popular with the great
mass of the people in a nation state, or that governments do
not often succeed in increasing their popularity by pursuing
an aggressive rather than a pacific policy. We feel the popularity of war and the ease with which the martial spirit of nations
can be stirred—the enthusiasm stimulated by the appeal to
force—is a basic fact that any complete theory of the cause
of war must be able to explain.

We cannot help thinking that those who hold this theory
must suppose that common people are fundamentally peaceful
and constructive and are only made warlike by the injustices
they suffer and the propaganda to which they are submitted.
We cannot accept this view. We do not think that the evidence
justifies the assumption that the exploited masses are simply
the tool of the exploiting classes—that common people are
kindly and friendly for the most part, and only bite when they
are deceived. We think the truer view to be—as we have
already stated—that the majority of human beings are prepared
to fight, that fighting is a form of behaviour fundamentally
natural to them, in situations and under stimuli the general
character of which is revealed by the inspection of the empirical
evidence that we have already carried out. While therefore
we see part of the truth in the view that nations fight for
economic advantages and elements of truth in the view that
the injustices and internal conflicts of a capitalist nation state
lead to war, we cannot feel that either view contains the
whole truth or that they can dispense with the prior analysis
of the causes of the willingness to fight.

What, then, are we to make of the doctrine ' that *nationalism*,
not capitalism, is the cause of war ? "

NATIONALISM AND WAR

Sometimes this theory appears to be no more than a statement that people now fight in groups that are called nations,

because it is obvious that they fought long before the modern
nation state had come into existence. If we are to make more
of this theory than a simple historical statement we must
suppose that those who hold this view are suggesting that the
fundamental loyalties and self-identifications of the individual
are now attached to the geographical and political group—
the nation—rather than to the social, economic, or ideological
groups in which the individual may at the same time find
himself placed. For recent times this is plainly true and it is
one of the main criticisms of Marx's views considered as a
theory of history. The dictum of the Communist Manifesto,
written in 1847–8 that ' National differences and antagonisms
between peoples are daily more and more vanishing . . .'
and that '. . . working men have no country,' make nonsense
now. His assumption that the development of capitalism would
make the loyalties felt by persons to their economic and social
classes supreme over all other loyalties has been completely
falsified. The last war found the great mass of the international (sic) proletariat loyal to their particular nation states
and not to the international brotherhood of working men.
Since the War the intensity of national loyalty has grown
rather than lessened. We live in an age of intense nationalism
and it is virtually certain therefore that future wars will be
fought between groups that are nations. All this is true and
important.

But the statement that ' nationalism is the cause of war '
cannot be regarded as a theory of the cause of war, but simply
as a descriptive or behaviourist generalization. To say that
people fight as nations does not explain why they fight at all.
It does not explain why group loyalties ever take an aggressive
form. As a theory of war it must suppose that it is obvious
that a group organization, once it is formed, will fight. It is
that prior problem that we have tried to resolve.

In terms of our own theory the true element in the view
that ' nationalism leads to war ' simply consists in recognizing
that the individual tends to identify himself with the predominant group of the age in which he lives. That is to say he
treats the events that happen to the group as though they
happened to him—as though the body of society were his
body. This process of identification—in part sensible and
objective and in part imaginative and false—accounts for the

intensity of group life. Without it the world would be a very different place and society a very different thing. But for the moment we are not concerned with the wider implications of this universal practice. We are concerned simply with the fact that many of the advantages and frustrations made an occasion for the use of force are found by the individual in the condition of, or events happening to, the group he sets first in his loyalties, whether it be feudal, national, or class. He transfers to the church or state or party his own loves and hatreds and treats the acquisitive opportunities and frustrations of the group as though they were possibilities or threats for him. Thus it is that in a religious age wars are fought by churches, in the age of organization in geographical and racial nations wars are fought between nations, and in any age in which international and inter-regional class organizations had triumphed, wars would be between classes. War is due to nationalism, not because the nation state is either a peacemaking or war-mongering form of organization in itself— there are pacific nations and aggressive nations—but because the triumph of aggressive impulses will always manifest itself in a group form and the great group organization of the age is the nation state.[1] And of course Marx may be right that the age in which we still live will be succeeded by an age in which class organizations and concomitant class war are the dominant phenomena of history.

Now if the theories that war is due to ' capitalism ' or ' nation-

---

[1] The argument and analysis of this section is particularly wide and general. To analyse in full the phenomenon of self-identification by the individual with the group and its implications for the study of politics would take us far beyond the limits of this article—even if the work had yet been done. All that we have attempted is the simplest application to the relations between aggressiveness and nationalism. It may be worth adding two short comments. (1) The phenomenon of identification with the group is far from simple. It does not mean that there is any universal tendency to feel at one with the existing regime. Persons hate the State as well as love it. Revolutionary parties pledged to kill the existing order can win majority support. But revolutionaries as much as patriots find personal significance to them—part reasonable, part exaggerated—in the condition of society. And in general it may be affirmed that the vast majority of human beings feel themselves strongly identified with the fortunes of some group outside themselves. Their own peaceful and aggressive impulses then find expression in group life in the ways that we have already discussed in Part I of the article. (2) The study of the way in which one group organization conquers another and becomes the dominant group of an age is one of the important tasks of history and sociology. We are only concerned with the problem of the aggressive and peaceful behaviour patterns common to all such organizations. We shall mention the problem of whether organizations differ in aggressiveness according to their form before we have finished.

alism ' are at best only half-truths, important consequences follow for the consideration of policy. We are not primarily concerned with the prevention of war in this article. That problem is dealt with in the remainder of the book. But it would be impossible to conclude what we have to say without mentioning the most pressing problem of our generation.

We cannot help feeling that if our interpretation of the evidence is correct—and we cannot help hoping that it is not—very little can be expected from some of the measures and policies proposed to-day. We would mention two in particular :

1. We do not see that much can be hoped from the abolition of capitalism or even the triumph of democracy. Neither of these institutional changes will remove or overcome the desire to appeal to force for the acquisition of advantages or the expression of transformed aggression and hatred. Whether such changes can cause or will accompany any diminution of transformed aggression itself we will discuss in a moment. In the meantime it is worth pointing out that democracies have often in fact been very aggressive. England has fought imperial wars of aggression. France, after a democratic revolution, overran Europe. We have, as yet, little experience of the supersession of capitalism, but what we have is not encouraging. Russia has not pursued an aggressive official foreign policy, but she has been exceedingly aggressive, until very recently,[1] against other nations by supporting revolutionary organizations within them. It is therefore not clear to us that a world of democracies, or a world of socialist dictatorships, or even a world of socialist democracies, would be wholly free from war.

2. Nor do we feel that much can be hoped, in the long run, from a weakening of loyalty to the nation group or a diminution of aggressive patriotism. The nation state is only the dominant group of this period. On empirical evidence alone, and assuming the continuity of human history, it is to be expected that this group loyalty will be replaced by another group loyalty just as fierce and just as dangerous to peace. Since religious loyalty gave place to national loyalty and international war appeared instead of religious war, so we should expect that in a new world devoid of nations, some other group

---

[1] Compare the change of front in the Third International in 1935.

would become the centre of transformed hatred and thus of war. This would seem certain unless something quite different had happened to change human character or unless some new institution had been created. Already it is said that in modern Europe a new kind of thing—an international alliance of nationalist fascisms—is coming to pass, foreshadowing future wars of political religion.

If little can be hoped from democracy or socialism, does that mean that there is no hope? Does the theory, that ' war is due to human nature ' hold the field with its gloomy scepticism over the existence or efficiency of any social therapy whatever? We think not. Some psychologists, impressed by the weight of their own evidence, have concluded so. We think that they are mistaken and that a more just appreciation of all the evidence indicates a method of procedure and a moderate hope of success.

III

If war is due to the fundamental aggressiveness of human beings, who tend to fight as individuals and in groups, then there are two solutions and two solutions only—either human beings must be changed or their aggressiveness must be restrained. Neither of these courses appear to us to be impracticable. To say that fighting has been a universal tendency in human behaviour in the past does not imply that it must always remain so in the future. People are what they are not only because of their inherited natures, but also because of the form of environment in which their inherited natures have developed. Hence it may be possible to change the character of adult behaviour by changing the environment in which our unchanged hereditary element develops. And, in a different way, it may be possible to ensure peace long before the slow process of individual change is complete.

Let us repeat at this point a simple fact that we have already twice affirmed. The preponderance of human impulses and inclinations has always been on the side of peaceful co-operation. Not only do the great majority of human beings spend the vast proportion of their time and energies in the constructive arts of peace, but almost always the greater part of the human race is in favour of preserving peace rather than permitting a resort to war. In both wars of recent history— that of Japan against Manchuria and of Italy against Abyssinia —nine-tenths of the nations of the world were opposed to the outbreak of war and were prepared to do something—though not enough—to preserve the peace. The reason for war is not the spontaneous aggressiveness of all mankind—if it were then indeed there would be little hope—but the ability of aggressive minorities to break the peace and by first taking up the sword to force everyone else to defend themselves in arms. War, like crime, is the result of the existence of anti-social minorities. But if war is due to minorities, cannot the majorities control them ? We wish to consider these two possibilities— of cure and of control—in turn.

EDUCATION AND WAR

It is our thesis that war is due to the expression in and through group life of the transformed aggressiveness of individuals. We therefore contend that to deal with the symptoms of transformed aggression—such as extreme nationalism, or class hatred—will not solve the problem of war. Aggression will only find another mode of expression. Is it, then, possible to deal with the cause ? Is it possible to diminish aggression itself ?

The immediate manifestations of transformed aggression is due, in our view, to the repression both by the self and by parental authority of simple aggression. Simple aggression, in its turn, we have argued, is due to the frustration of impulse. It would seem upon this analysis that adult aggressiveness could be diminished either by a reduction in the repression of simple aggression or by a reduction in the extent to which impulse is frustrated. If children could be frustrated less frequently— given more open access to the means of their satisfaction— or if they were punished less severely when they resented frustration ; if, in short, they were allowed to express desire and anger more freely it should follow, contrary to common expectation, that they would make more happy, more peaceful, and more social adults. The evidence shows overwhelmingly, as we have already seen, that the suppression of simple aggression does not kill it. It drives it underground and makes it far more horrible and destructive. It is only in the expression of it that it becomes diminished. It is only within the circumstances of freedom that social habits and a spontaneous desire to co-operate can flourish and abound. 'Spare the rod and spoil the child'—as a quiet and convenient member of the familial group. Spare the rod and make a free, independent, friendly, and generous adult human being.

There are three points to be made in amplification of this suggestion :

1. A certain amount of frustration is inevitable and a certain amount of external repression is almost equally so. A child cannot have all that it wants. In the first place the parents may not be rich enough to supply it even with enough to eat. In the second place some of its desires—though we suspect they would be few except in the first few years of life—are contradictory and dangerous. A baby must be denied the fire that it wishes to reach or the bright but poisonous berry that it wishes to suck. In the third place the satisfaction of some of its desires may make social life impossible or intolerable. The child cannot rampage when its parents are tired or ill. It cannot be taken for a walk when its mother must get the tea. Upon a thousand occasions frustration is inevitable. But we suggest that even if frustration is inevitable it should be reduced to a minimum and could be reduced enormously below its present level. The restraint of impulse is so frequently carried out upon principle—as a desirable form of 'discipline.' Parents believe that children ought not to have what they want—that denial of impulse will make a good character. We hold that the opposite of this is the truth.

Nevertheless, some frustration is inevitable. What then can be done to alleviate its ill effects ? We suggest that much more can be done by refusing to suppress and punish the natural resentment that frustration calls forth. This we feel to be the essential point. Take the child away from the fire, refuse to take it for a walk, deny it a second piece of cake, but avoid being angry or hurt or disapproving if a scream of rage or a kick on the shins is the immediate consequence of thwarting the child's will to happiness. To permit children to express their *feelings* of aggression whilst preventing *acts* of irremediable destruction is, we suggest, one of the greatest gifts that parents can give to their children.

2. We believe the evidence suggests that such methods of

education will have consequences precisely the opposite of those expected by the parent unaware of the evidence of modern analytical psychology. People greatly under-estimate the rapidity and strength with which the social and affectionate impulses of the free child develop. And yet it is blindness to do so. After all, enormous advantages accrue to the child from co-operation. It is, as we have emphasized *ad nauseam*, the overwhelming impulse of human life. And we suggest that the child, freed from frustration and unsympathetic discipline, will in fact become the very opposite of the popular picture of the ' spoiled child.' Instead of violent and un-governable anger, inordinate selfishness, and vanity, the child that is not afraid to express its feelings is likely to exhibit affection, independence, sociability, and courage more rapidly and more naturally than a repressed child. Such children, we suggest, become reasonable and sociable at a surprisingly early age. Familial life with them is not a nightmare of disorder, or the false calm of strong discipline, but a moderately peaceful and very lively society of free, equal, and willing co-operation.

3. At the same time we do not wish to over-draw the picture. There are certain inevitable conflicts and sources of disturbance in individual and familial life. Sexual jealousy for one thing is unavoidable. It seems unlikely to us that the strain between father and son, mother and daughter, can be wholly avoided. Nor does the reduction of external repression remove internal conflict. Self-repression—the fear that anger felt towards the source of satisfaction will ' kill the goose that lays the golden eggs '—will still remain. Hence the reduction of repression is not a panacea. It will not produce a familial heaven or a race of perfect adults in a generation. Neurosis and aggressiveness will still be there. Social friction and the threat to peace will not be wholly eliminated. We only suggest that these things will be greatly reduced.

This doctrine is somewhat more speculative than our analysis of the causes of aggressiveness. It is not established by the existing evidence with the same degree of certainty. The number of children educated more freely is still small. No society has embarked upon the experiment of a wide and rapid change in the technique of parental control. No generation has yet grown up that has been influenced by

D

the spread of these ideas. It is, therefore, too soon to say whether a change in the educational environment can bring about a substantial reduction in the aggressiveness of adults. We personally feel that the evidence gathered from the treatment of children is overwhelmingly on one side. We believe it to be almost certain that if children were actually brought up more freely they would be much happier, much more reasonable, and much more sociable.[1] We think it obvious that social and international relations would greatly benefit if people were happier, more reasonable and more sociable. But this belief is still in the realm of probability rather than fact. It is, of course, a purely empirical question. Will a certain form of education make human adults less aggressive without making them less strong? It is the combination of strength with reasonableness, of power with affection, that we think desirable. We have no faith in, nor desire to educate, a pacifist generation. We believe that the rejection of force, and the passive acceptance of other people's aggression, to be as profoundly neurotic as the manifestation of transformed aggression itself. But with the subject of pacifism we are not concerned. Its logic, though not its psychological origin, is dealt with in the next paper. We only wish to emphasize that what we do not expect is a generation of persons unable or unwilling to protect themselves, who kneel down before the aggressor and fling wide their gates to his attack, to arise from a better form of emotional education, but a generation of men and women who will defend their rights and yet willingly concede equal rights to others, who will accept the judgment of third parties in the resolution of disputes, who will neither bully nor eat humble pie, who will fight, but only in defence of law, who are willing and friendly members of a positive and just society.

Unfortunately this hope is not for us but only for generations that shall come long after us. We have not the time nor opportunity to do these things. It would take generations to affect the course of international relations by emotional education. And, in any case, there is not the remotest possibility of beginning now. Half the nations of the world are in the grip of regimes in which this type of education, so far from

---

[1] The evidence of the therapeutic value of analysing aggressive children—a process consisting amongst other things of treating them more sympathetically and without punishment—is particularly convincing on this point.

being encouraged, is being destroyed. Even in democratic communities there is no widespread belief in the kind of argument we have been advocating—much less is there any serious attempt to reform familial practice in this direction. Even if there were, the successful execution of a new technique of parental guidance requires a new and less neurotic generation to carry it through. Improvement in the emotional atmosphere that surrounds the representative child can only be brought about slowly and from generation to generation as each group of parents brings to its children a less warped and aggressive personality. It is possible to begin but not to proceed rapidly with this basic social therapy. In the meantime, if this is all the hope there is we shall have perished by half a dozen wars. And each war, by strengthening the fears and hatreds inside national groups, will make the task of better education more difficult. Is there then no hope except for generations centuries hence and parts of the world far removed from Western Europe? We think this to be a false conclusion and we are thus brought to a consideration of the use of force to preserve peace.

GOVERNMENT AND COLLECTIVE SECURITY

Our theory implies among many other important things for the study of society, a theory of the value of government. Just as the greater part of human endeavour is directed to the purposes of peace, so the main activity of government is the organization of peaceful co-operation. Whatever our theory of the state may be, it cannot be denied that most of its labour is devoted to the organization of peaceful activities and defining, without the use of force, the framework of laws and institutions within which individuals and smaller groups can work together in tranquillity. But the State has another and vitally important task. In all modern societies—whether democratic or dictatorial, capitalist or communist—the government and the apparatus of force that it controls seeks to prevent the breakdown of social equilibrium into civil war. One of the worst crimes in any State is treason against it, and the vast and increasing power of the State is built up to crush the various aggressive minorities who propose to resort to force in defiance of the law.

There is no pacifism within the State. If members of the criminal minority resort to force, force will be used against them. If larger groups threaten the peace by rioting, first the police and then the more heavily armed forces at the disposal of the Government will be used against them. The theory and practice of government is the theory and practice of mobilizing an overwhelming force against anyone or any group that will not keep the law in peace. In our view it is therefore not surprising that the area of the strong nation state has been predominantly the area of peace. Of course, this is not always so. Civil war has broken out more than once in the strongest modern states. But almost all wars and all the largest wars have been between nations—that is, in the realm of anarchy outside the rule of law supported by force.

No doubt there exists another great force making for peace within the State—that is, the spontaneous acceptance of law and the moral sanction that law *qua* law therefore possesses. Peace is preserved and the law obeyed in the vast majority of cases without the direct intervention or supervision of the police. Yet force is, nevertheless, present in the background. People may often obey the law because they wish to. But they must obey it whether they wish to or not—or go to prison. And, in fact, there is always a criminal minority who do not obey the law against whom force always is and must be used. There is always a disruptive tendency present in society—a tendency to form aggressive and revolutionary minorities—and, if and when they are allowed to grow without the opposition of force, society draws nearer and nearer to civil war. The recent history of Europe offers many examples of such a development. Moreover, it seems easy to us to exaggerate the strength of the feeling for the moral authority of the law. It seems straining the use of terms to say that the dissident minorities of authoritarian governments ' accept the law.' It seems plainly untrue that peasants admit the moral sanctity of oppressive systems of agrarian law or that the organized proletariat of a capitalist system really *accept* the justice of the present laws of property. It may be that they feel that an unjust law is better than no law at all, but few dictators, at any rate, would willingly divorce themselves from the use of force and expect internal peace to be preserved by the strength of moral sentiment alone.

Although it is well outside the subject of this article and constitutes an altogether larger question, the authors cannot help feeling that the existing evidence largely supports the view that while there is no unbreakable link between peace and justice there is such a connection between peace and force. In their view, peace has often existed in the past, and exists in many places now, where the general condition of society is not accepted as just. It is tolerated because the alternative to it—the appeal to force—has been made a less eligible alternative. We believe that some persons and groups are so aggressive that, in the absence of force to restrain them, they will break the peace and compel everyone else, reluctantly but sensibly, to arm themselves in order to resist force with force and thus escape arbitrary and unscrupulous evil thrust upon them by unjust means. Peace can only triumph with a sword in its hand. Such is the commonplace view of all intelligent supporters of international law.

The application of this view to international affairs and the problem of international war is obvious. Article XVI of the Covenant of the League of Nations was and is, in our view, the only hope for the *peace* of the world. Until law is backed by force there seems to us no hope for law or peace. Law is not justice, but neither is war. Aggressive minorities will make war, but they will not make justice. And while the achievement of justice will greatly aid the establishment of peace, the handing over of the world to the will of the minority of aggressive states will secure neither justice nor peace. Thus, while the struggle for justice and for a system of law that is sufficiently just to be accepted freely by all men is one of the central tasks before this generation, the evidence suggests to the present writers most strongly that the organization of international force for the preservation of international peace and the fulfilment of international law is the most urgent task of all.

Of course, force will not cure the impulses of aggression. Some psychologists, so impressed by this fact and also by the consideration that government is a symbol to most people of their own projected conscience, have concluded that the organization of force is not favourable to peace. We should agree that force is not a therapeutic agent. A policeman will not cure a murderer of the desire to kill. An international air force will not cure Hitler or Mussolini of the desire to kill. But that, we feel, is not the point. The immediate problem is not to cure the aggressor, but to prevent the aggression, or to see if the aggression takes place it can only lead to one outcome—the vindication of the law. That is the vital point —the problem is to see that the great majority of human beings who are peaceful and the great majority of human activity that is constructive should be protected from the savage and destructive violence of the aggressive minorities. It is only if the lovers of peace and social reconstruction will use force to protect themselves that peace within and without the nation state can be preserved.

Thus, as we see it, there are two ways and only two in which war can be reduced in its frequency and violence—one slow, curative, and peaceful, aimed at the removal of the ultimate causes of war in human character by a new type of emotional education—the other immediate, coercive, and aimed at symptoms, the restraint of the aggressor by force.

CONCLUSION

This brings us to the end of what we have to say. We have pursued a very restricted theme. It has not been possible to consider the psychological evidence in detail. The vast anthropological material has scarcely been touched. We have not traced out in detail the classification of the historical occasion of wars into our categories of simple and more complex aggressiveness. All this urgently needs doing. Nor have we considered the application of our views to the other problems of social behaviour. We hope at some future date to attempt some of these tasks.

One of our omissions is particularly marked and serious. We have failed to consider the question whether certain types of institution or patterns of society stimulate or alleviate the fundamental tendencies to aggressiveness in children and adults. Does democracy or socialism or a peasant economy— or any other form of society—make in itself, for peace? We have argued explicitly that one kind of institution—the pattern of emotional education current in society—is quite vital in this respect. We are inclined very tentatively to suggest that that is the most important single institution.

Yet certain other simple correlations are probably observable. On the whole and speaking very roughly it would, we suppose, be true to say that democratic peoples, and peoples in the democratic periods of their history, are less aggressive than authoritarian peoples and periods. It may very well be that Socialist democracy would be less aggressive still. But it seems to us that this correlation of democracy and equality on the one hand with peace on the other is less likely to be a correlation of cause and effect as of the parallel effects of a common cause. We are inclined to think, that is to say, that the kind of people who can support the responsibility, freedom, and toleration required by democracy are also likely to be peaceful. They are not peaceful because they are democratic. They are peaceful and democratic because they are the kind of people they are. And the same argument we feel would apply to any correlation between equality and peacefulness. But this whole question of the relation between the emotional character of the individual and the group on the one hand and its social institutions on the other is far too vast a field to consider here. We can only state our belief that the most important and fruitful possibilities in contemporary social studies lie in the further exploration of this field—the borderland between individual psychology and the study of comparative social institutions.

To conclude—we believe that the study of the causal relation between personal aggressiveness and war throws a flood of light upon a universal phenomenon in history—the willingness of groups to fight. We think it reconciles the traditional and pessimistic view that war is due to the unalterable characteristics of ' human nature ' with the exaggerated and recently disappointed expectations of the post-war generation in which we grew up. We think the evidence suggests that war is an endemic but not an incurable disease of human society. We think it reveals a long period therapeutic policy. It seems to us to reinforce abundantly the conclusion that a strong organ of collective security is the only possible protection from war. It throws into sharp relief the great tragedy of the present decade—that the democratic and peace-loving nations of Europe seem to have missed through an infirmity of purpose and a love of sovereignty the opportunity to unite themselves in strength for the defence of law and the protection of peace. We have written in the hope that the analysis of this evidence may help some future generation, who, rising once more from a surfeit of hatred and destruction, may perhaps ask with more sober hope and with more scientific realism—can we prevent this thing from happening again ?

E. F. M. D.

APPENDIX

AN EXAMINATION OF THE PSYCHOLOGICAL AND ANTHROPOLOGICAL EVIDENCE

In this article it has been contended that, since war is a particular example of the widespread animal activity of fighting, a scientific study of fighting should and does throw light upon the origin of war. It is now proposed to describe some of the observations upon which we have built our theory of war. First an attempt will be made to review the evidence at present available regarding individual acts of aggression. An attempt will be made to answer the questions : On what occasions do individuals fight? What about? And to what purpose?

In the second part a few observations regarding group aggression are described. They are deliberately selected with the object of demonstrating that group aggressions are not always explicable in ordinary rational terms and are often only to be understood by reference to the more complicated psychological theories arrived at by a study of individuals. The examples given are too few to do more than illustrate our general contention that the study of individual aggression is indispensable to a proper understanding of group aggression.

It is true that we believe that the motives which produce war in Melanesia and persecution in Germany are extremely widespread and influence profoundly all international relations. We believe indeed that international relations are incomprehensible and inexplicable if these motives are not constantly considered. Nevertheless we are aware that our few examples constitute no proof, and that our belief in the importance of these forces can only be substantiated by more far-reaching and thorough researches than have as yet been attempted.

A. STUDIES OF INDIVIDUAL AGGRESSION

(1) THE SOCIAL LIFE OF MONKEYS AND APES

The science of comparative social psychology has made important advances of recent years. It is not long since our knowledge of animal societies depended entirely upon traveller's tales and the random observations of naturalists. Sometimes these are accurate, but there is usually bias, almost always anthropomorphic. Recent work, however, has done much to correct this tendency and to put the subject upon a more scientific basis.

Zuckermann's study of the social life of mammals, with special reference to monkeys and apes,[1] is a particularly valuable contribution in the wide biological background which it affords for the study of human sociology. Unlike insects, whose societies are sometimes quoted, sub-human primates are nearly related to man and are identical in fundamental physiological processes. Moreover, observation has shown that in certain important respects the social life of monkeys and apes is more like that of man than it is like that of other mammals. For these reasons the authors believe Zuckermann's observations on peace and war amongst baboons are of real value in understanding the problems of peace and war amongst humans.[2]

Before considering the special problem of aggression in apes, it may be as well to discuss the structure of their social life in comparison with that of other mammals.

Zuckermann contends that the forces which influence the congregation of mammals into groups are of two kinds, firstly, an ecological (or geographical) factor and secondly, the nature of their sexual and parental instincts. The ecological factor has been seriously underestimated in the past. It is simply the natural partiality which animals of the same species will have for a certain type of environment. There is an optimum climate and food supply for each given species and each individual of that species will want to live where it can be found. It seems likely that such ecological forces are responsible for the dramatic group migrations of certain birds and animals and for the tendency of grazing animals to move in herds and carnivores to live further apart from each other. Ecological forces in fact explain most of what was formerly put down to the operations of a herd instinct.

But they are of little help in explaining the relations subsisting between individuals within a herd. These can only

[1] Zuckermann, *The Social Life of Monkeys and Apes*, London, 1932.
[2] No doubt systematic observations on the social life and aggressive behaviour of the mammals such as dogs, cats, and horses would also be valuable, but, as is described later, their social life differs in important respects from that of man, and furthermore it would be impossible to do the data justice in the space at our disposal.

be understood in psychological and physiological terms. Zuckermann has demonstrated that they depend almost entirely upon the mating and breeding peculiarities of each species.[1] For purposes of sociological analysis he divides mammals into three main groups according to their mating habits.

(1) Mammals who have a mating season and a quiescent (anoestrous) period. In these the social group endures only so long as its members are sexually potent. Some of them like the jaguar spend the anoestrous in solitude. The seals spend it in separate male and female herds. Rabbits on the other hand mix together during the anoestrous period but their social life remains asexual. A few species such as the horse maintain a familial grouping during part of the period, but in none of them is the sexual link maintained until the next mating season.

(2) In the second group are mammals who, whilst having no special season of the year for mating, mate only when the female is on heat. As in the first group the sexual link between male and female is constantly being broken and remade. There is no permanent union between male and female and the family consists only of mother and young. There is no father in the social sense.[2]

(3) Primates (monkeys, apes and humans) are unique inasmuch as the female will mate at any time and both male and female are always sexually active to some extent. Anoestrous periods are unknown. As a result there is a permanent heterosexual interest which holds the sexes together in permanent sexual associations and the family consists not only of mother and young. The male retains possession of his female or females, has frequent intercourse with them all the year round, and consequently is a father socially as well as biologically.

The monkeys and apes therefore have a social life altogether different from that of the lower mammals, but identical in basic structure to that of man. For this reason it is to be expected that the study of the social life of subhuman primates will be of value and relevance for understanding certain problems of human social life. But before examining the fighting which occurs in monkey communities it may be as well to consider in more detail their mode of existence.

---

[1] 'It is impossible to define animal social relationships other than those of sexual male and female, and nursing female and offspring.' Op. cit.

[2] Apparent 'faithfulness' between male and female in periodically mating animals is probably the combined result of proximity and chance.

As above indicated the primates are distinguished from other mammals in having social ties of a considerable degree of permanency. The family—husband, wives and children—is the unit. The male retains possession of his females because he is in constant need of them and other males are commonly regarded as potential enemies. No other male except the overlord enters into sexual relations with the females of a family group. Since some males have more than one wife, many monkeys and apes are therefore forced to live either temporarily or permanently in celibacy. This is spent in a variety of ways according to the species. Some become the ' lone males ' that are occasionally encountered. Others form bachelor clubs and go about in male bands. Still others, like the baboons, join up with a family party, though remaining on strictly platonic terms with the females.

The family groups also vary in their sociability with others. In some species it is rare to meet with more than one or two families together. But in others large troops are formed by the union of numerous family parties and their attendant bachelors.

The existence of these larger communities needs explanation. No doubt economic and climatic (ecological) conditions play an important part. Where conditions are bad and food is scarce there will be isolated groups consisting of only one family, where conditions are better bigger groups, each of many families, will gather. The formation of such larger groups may be purely ecological in origin, but there are grounds for believing that psychological forces are also at work. For instance, a sexual interest in the mates of others and the possibility of acquiring more wives is likely to draw bachelors and families together.[1] Whether the advantages of co-operation play a part is uncertain. Naturalists have so tended to exaggerate it in the past that caution is required in examining evidence.[2] But there can be no doubt that co-opera-

---

[1] ' This constant attraction of the females for the males may also be one explanation of the occurrence of large hordes of monkeys, the females of harems attracting to their vicinity both unattached males and the males of other family parties, even though there is no overt expression of heterosexual interest except within the family.' (Op. cit., p. 214.)

[2] ' Many accounts have been published in which reference is made to sentinels placed by baboons during their foraging and pillaging activities. The use of the term ' sentinel ' is altogether unjustifiable. There is no evidence of any kind that special members of a troop are placed on its outskirts for the specific purpose of " doing sentry-go," and so far as can be observed, any baboon of a pack who happens to see an approaching human being will bark.' (Op. cit., p. 206.)

On the other hand the fact that species of primates which come closest into contact with man and pillage his farms are those which live in bands of several families, suggests that there may be some primitive co-operation in attack.

tion, if present at all, is very little developed, and of no such vital importance as it has become in human societies. For baboon families split off and rejoin the multifamilial groups indiscriminately with the result that the groups have neither stability nor government.

With this analysis of the social background in the life of apes it is possible to understand the circumstances in which fighting occurs amongst them.

Zuckermann's observations were made principally upon a community of baboons kept in captivity at the London Zoo and checked by observations on groups in other zoos and also in their wild state in South Africa. The unnatural conditions of captivity probably made considerable differences of degree in the behaviour of the animals, but observations of their wild state suggest that it was normal in kind.[1] By far the most frequent origin of a serious fight was over the possession of wives. For weeks or even months the community would live in comparative peace, the family groups remaining together and the residual bachelors either forming mutual attachments or living platonically with a family. But such peaceful social life on occasion broke up into pandemonium, resulting in gruesome and bitter fights in which the whole community was involved. One of the worst was when thirty females were added to the group in an attempt to make the ratio of the sexes more even. The result was disastrous. A fierce fight for their possession broke out and, perhaps due to the restrictive surroundings, within a month no less than half the imported females had been killed. This is Zuckermann's account :

'On 27 June 1927, two years after the Hill was founded, the existing population' (consisting of fifty-six animals, only five or six of which were female) 'was . . . augmented by thirty adult females and five immature males. . . . The new arrivals stirred the Hill into great excitement, and all the old males tried to secure females, fifteen of whom were killed in the fights that occurred between the 27 July and the end of August. These fights are definitely sexual in

---

[1] ' It is also possible that captive conditions modify fighting behaviour. Confined to a small area animals cannot separate from one another as they would in a natural environment. A baboon worsted in a fight is unable to escape from aggressors. An animal not dominant enough to maintain himself and his harem in a large herd cannot succeed in retaining his females by avoiding contact with his fellows, as he might in a wild state.

'These considerations suggest that fights may often be carried much further in captivity than they would be in nature. This, however, adds to their interest. From the point of view of the observer, confinement concentrates a normal response both temporally and spatially.' (Op. cit., p. 217.)

nature. The males fight for the females, who are usually fatally injured in the mêlée which rages around them.'[1]

It is obvious that this fight was provoked by the unnatural conjunction of numerous unmated males and females. But the fights which followed the death of a husband or the attempted abduction of a wife would presumably occur also in the wild. Fights over the possession of widows were of regular occurrence.

' Early in 1927 a young female was killed the day after three males had died. In February 1928 a male, whose body showed the scars of recent fights, died of pneumonia : four days after its death a male was killed, and two days later a second animal died from injuries. On two separate occasions in 1929 a female was killed in less than a week after the death of a male, and in 1930 one female was killed within four days of the death of another. The number of fatal fights that have followed deaths on the Hill is too great to be without significance, and the meaning of the cor-relation is obvious. The equilibrium of a social group is dependent upon the mutual reactions of all its members. The death of any single individual upsets the state of balance, and fighting commonly breaks out before a new equilibrium is reached.'[2]

Attempts to abduct females were another frequent cause of fights which would presumably also occur in the wild.

' . . . early in 1929, the population of the Hill was forty-one males, four of which were immature, and nine females, one of which was nursing the young animal that was born in October 1928. These nine females were owned by eight males, there being seven " monogamous " family parties and one that was " bigamous." These relationships were stable. With little exception there was no promiscuity. Five of the nine females lost their lives in fights caused by other males attempting their abduction.'[3]

Such abductions usually start ' as a quarrel between two animals. There is no evidence that it begins as a concerted attack of unmated males upon the harem.'[4]

' The normal behaviour of most unmated male baboons suggests their passive indifference to the presence of females

[1] Op. cit., pp. 218 and 219.   [2] Op. cit., pp. 221–222.
[3] Op. cit., p. 225.   [4] Op. cit., p. 253.

within the colony. On rare occasions, however, the atmosphere suddenly changes and every male appears to be trying, at the peril of life, to secure a female in an attack upon a harem. The behaviour of one male influences another, and there have been few " sexual fights " on Monkey Hill in which most members of the colony have not been engaged. Though mated animals have never been known to initiate a " sexual fight," almost all of them have been observed participating once such a fight has begun. The " sexual fights " on Monkey Hill have been so serious that they have been responsible for the deaths of thirty female baboons.[1] After each of the serious fights had ended in the death of the female round which it raged, the colony settled down in a state of balance which as subsequent events proved, contained all the seeds of further disruption.'[2]

The tendency for small fights to draw into their ambit large numbers of originally uninterested individuals was shown also in the numerous minor scuffles which occurred. Although no lethal battles took place, except those over the possession of wives, hardly a day passed without a scuffle between the bachelors.

'. . . it is often difficult to understand the causes of their quarrels. Occasionally it is due to a baboon attempting to secure food that is snatched by a more dominant fellow. Sometimes a fight is precipitated by one animal rushing to attack another who has evoked a squeal of terror from an immature animal. Usually, however, fights are begun as a display of dominance, one animal suddenly threatening any other in its vicinity. The aggressive baboon begins to grind its teeth, to ' yawn ', to grimace, and stare at the enemy it has chosen, while it makes quick thrusting movements on the rocks with its hand. The response to such behaviour is almost reflex in character. The threatened animal, either alone or together with its neighbours, begins a reciprocal display of dominance. Once two are involved in such a quarrel, it is rare for others not to participate. They rush to the scene, generally joining the animal who is at the

---

[1] ' Of the thirty-three females that died, thirty lost their lives in fights, in which they were the prizes fought for by the males. . . .' ' It is difficult to believe that so large a proportion of females would be killed in a natural community, even though there can be no doubt that wild female baboons are also exposed to the attacks of their fellows. Thus scars were seen on practically every carcass of an adult female baboon that I obtained in South Africa. . . .'

[2] Op. cit., p. 252.

moment less dominant. Sometimes the disturbance spreads throughout the colony and mated males and their family parties join in the fight. The more aggressive animal seems to be unaffected by the increase in the number of the enemies he has called upon himself, and thus the baboon fight assumes its peculiar character of a single animal defending himself against a group. . . . It is rare for these scuffles to develop into fights in which the animals seriously hurt one another, the aggressive animal usually routing the group he opposes.'[1]

Zuckermann discusses the question of dominance at length, showing how the comparative stability of the group depends upon the recognition on the part of the weaker animals of the superiority of the stronger. When a previously dominant animal is challenged a fight ensues.

' Fundamentally, females are also treated as material objects, and are secured by the more dominant animals, the weaker males remaining unmated. In a baboon colony an animal may be dominant so far as females are concerned, whereas his dominance may not be exhibited at feeding times. An overlord may scuffle with bachelors for the possession of some fruit and may be worsted. He does not, however, thus lose caste, nor do such circumstances usually lead to serious fighting. If, on the other hand, adult bachelors were to try to steal his female, the situation would immediately result in serious fighting. If the bachelors are routed in such a fight, the overlord maintains his dominant position within the herd. If, on the other hand, he is dispossessed, he immediately loses caste, to become submissive to those animals whom he formerly dominated.'[2]

The fact that no serious battles occurred over the possession of food is of importance, especially when, as will be seen, this is also found to be true of many primitive human societies. Of course it is not known for certain what happens in wild communities of baboons. The fact that there were no serious fights over food in the London Zoo may only be a tribute to the diet provided in captivity. It is possible that in harder circumstances rivalry for food might constitute as serious a cause of fighting as rivalry over females. Nevertheless what evidence is available points to sexual rivalry as the sole cause of serious fighting amongst baboons.

¹ Op. cit., p. 249.   ² Op. cit., pp. 235–236.

Relevance of this Evidence for Human Society.

Many arguments may be brought to prove that this evidence is not only irrelevant to the topic of war, but actually misleading because baboons differ in many respects from humans. Even if baboons do behave like this, it might be argued, that is no proof that there are any such proclivities in man. No one likes to think that there are in himself such violent propensities ; we are all anxious to prove that we are pacific even if others are not. Yet there is evidence to suggest that mankind is not so different from the baboons after all and that men will fight for the possession of wives like any monkey.

In the first place some of the simplest peoples live in societies identical in structure to those of baboons. ' Among the lower gatherers we generally hear of quite small groups, two or three to five or six families in the usual sense of that term making perhaps two "enlarged families" of brothers or possibly cousins with their wives, children, and grandchildren.'[1] Like baboons they have no government or authority and like baboons a frequent source of fighting is over the abduction of women.

Amongst rather more advanced peoples who have attained to some degree of organization sexual rivalry remains a source of conflict. ' Nearly all the native fights in Australia are over women. The abduction of women, rape, elopement, and the refusal to surrender a girl promised in marriage are the commonest causes. In Central Australia intertribal quarrels arise chiefly from wife-stealing, although not infrequently the elopement of a woman with a man of another group is a cause of serious trouble between the two groups.' ' The Greenlanders who have no war, nevertheless occasionally quarrel among themselves, and "women and love are among the most frequent causes of bloodshed." The Chinook Indians were likewise peaceably inclined, but were frequently involved in quarrels resulting it is said, "from the abduction of women more frequently than from other causes." '[2]

English seamen of a century ago were not radically different as the history of Pitcairn's Island Colony shows.[3] In 1790 nine English seamen, mutineers of H.M.S. *Bounty*, landed on Pitcairn's Island together with six men and eleven women

---

[1] Hobhouse, Wheeler, and Ginsberg, *The Material Culture and Social Institutions of the Simpler Peoples.*

[2] Davie, *The Evolution of War*, Yale University Press, 1929, p. 99.

[3] This account is taken from the material collected by H. L. Shapiro in *The Heritage of the Bounty*, Gollancz, 1936.

whom they had brought with them from Tahiti. They were a friendly group. The Englishmen were fleeing from justice with their native wives whom they had picked up during a stay in Tahiti, whilst the native men accompanied them in a spirit of adventure. Pitcairn's Island was chosen for colonization because it was uninhabited and difficult of access. A successful landing was made, huts built and agriculture begun. Although the Englishmen decided to partition the land equally amongst themselves, making the natives their virtual slaves, no serious dissension arose, and the colony remained peaceful and industrious for the first two years.

The first dispute arose over a woman. One of the Englishmen early lost his wife in an accident, she falling over a cliff whilst collecting eggs. After a while he became dissatisfied with his celibate life and decided to sail off to another island to look for a wife. Since he was a useful artisan, his companions were reluctant to see him go. They consequently approached one of the two married natives and arranged for him to make over his wife to the English widower. The natives were incensed by this treatment, and from having been the friends and later the servants of the Englishmen they became their serious enemies. Their plot to murder the Englishmen was discovered, however, and instead the English murdered two of them.

Another two years elapsed before the natives again became dissatisfied. It is difficult to know precisely what precipitated this quarrel, but apparently cruelty from two of the whites was partly to blame. On this occasion the Tahitian's plot was more successful and five of the nine Englishmen were killed and the remainder driven to the far end of the island. The natives then proceeded to fight amongst themselves for the choice of the dead men's wives. One of them was killed in this fight and another was killed by a native woman in revenge for her dead husband. The Englishmen then attacked and killed the remaining two native men.

Of the fifteen men who had landed only four, all English, thus remained alive after four years. After one had drunk himself to death, a final murder was committed. Another accident bereft one of the three remaining men of his wife. Instead of selecting another from the now surplus supply of women, he insisted with threats that the only woman who would suit him was the wife of one of the others. He became so menacing that the other two decided that in self-defence they had best kill him. They consequently murdered him in his sleep. One of the remaining two men died soon afterwards from natural causes, leaving a single white man, nine native women, and twenty-five children. Thenceforward peace reigned supreme under a benevolent patriarch, who, afflicted by a sense of sin, became increasingly religious.

Thus within ten years twelve out of fifteen men had been murdered. Two of the fights occurred as a result of successful or attempted abduction. Whether sexual jealousy was operative in beginning the biggest fight is obscure, but once begun rivalry for the possession of wives prolonged it.

Conclusions.

The main conclusions to be drawn from this evidence may be summarized.

(1) The basic biological forces binding individual animals into social groups are ecological and sexual. The particular form of society characteristic of each species depends upon the interplay of these factors which vary for each species. Forces such as vicarious sexual interest and the advantage of co-operation may play subsidiary roles.

(2) The primates are alone amongst mammals in that the sexual tie is not constantly broken and remade. The females become the permanent property of the males who retain possession by force, and the family—husband, wives and children—is the basic social unit.

(3) Many of the primates live in large groups, each consisting of a number of families and bachelors, knit together by loose bonds. There are daily scuffles over food and displays of dominance, but serious fights only occur at intervals of weeks or even months.

(4) The only serious fights known to occur in baboon communities centre round the possession of females. They begin either when there is an unmated female available, through death of a husband or other cause, or else with the attempted abduction of a wife by an unmated male. Such fights frequently end in the death of the prize and sometimes also of some of the males.

(5) Fights usually begin between two males but they always become general, every male in the community attempting to obtain possession of one or more females.

(6) Comparative equilibrium is not restored until all the females have become the permanent and undisputed property of individual males.

(7) The evidence suggests that when man lives in unorganized groups, he tends towards a social life basically similar to that of apes. The main social ties are sexual and familial.

(8) Human groups of this kind are hardly more peaceful than baboon societies. Fighting breaks out sporadically, alternating with peaceful periods.

(9) Although there may be various causes of fighting, it appears that, as in baboons, one of its principal sources is over the possession of wives.

(10) The evidence in fact supports Hobbes' view that without government and in a state of nature, man's life, thanks to his animal passions and rivalries, tends to be ' solitary, poor, nasty, brutish, and short '.

(2) SOCIAL DEVELOPMENT AND AGGRESSION IN CHILDREN

Further light on the forces influencing human social life is shed by the study of children. Children are usually more direct and more honest in their expression of feeling than adults, with the result that a true estimate of their real motives is easier to obtain. Conclusions regarding adult societies, drawn from the study of children, rest on the observation that many forces present in childhood continue active in adult life.

Several valuable studies of the development of personal relations in children have been carried out. Those based on psycho-analytic technique are considered in the next section. Of the less controversial studies based on direct observation that of Dr. Susan Isaacs is the most comprehensive.[1] Much that follows is derived from her book which describes the work and play of a group of small children in a comparatively unrestricted environment. Once again before considering the incidence of aggression in these children it may be well to discuss the forces making for social unity and peace.

The chief additional factor not found amongst apes which binds children into social groups is co-operation. It seems sometimes to be thought that children would never become either sociable or co-operative if they were not taught to be. This is certainly untrue. Many observations go to show that happy children develop into sociable and co-operative beings as spontaneously as they learn to walk or talk. Nevertheless the development of these abilities takes time and like any other natural function may be interfered with. Isaacs recognizes three phases through which a normal child passes in its progress from selfish solitude to sociable co-operation.

(1) Up to two or three years the small child ignores other children and plays almost entirely by himself or perhaps with

---

[1] Isaacs, *Social Development in Young Children*, Routledge, 1933.

an adult. In this stage of solitary play co-operation is non-existent.

(2) After about three years comes a dawning recognition of the presence of other children, but still no true group is formed. Each child in this phase behaves independently, *making use* of others to further his own ends, but failing utterly to appreciate that others have ends also. It is assumed that the other person will behave exactly as it is wished they should, the possibility of their also having wishes being ignored.

(3) It is not until the age of at least four and often later that a gradual adjustment to the true social situation occurs. Slowly the personalities and independent purposes of others are appreciated. Common ends come to be envisaged and joint action in their attainment undertaken. Moreover it becomes possible for a child to sacrifice his own immediate ends for later advantages. He is willing to become the other fellow's wheelbarrow for a time in order later to enlist another soldier in his army. The principle of ' give and take ' develops.

But such temporary abrogation of wishes is extremely difficult for many children. It requires great trust in the goodwill of the others and it is not therefore surprising that the more fearful the child the less co-operative he is. Anything which causes him to believe that the other children are selfish and grasping will naturally make co-operation with them impossible. Unfortunately, as will be discussed in the next section, the human mind has a great capacity for seeing and exaggerating hostility and greed in others. As a result co-operation develops with difficulty and in many people remains precarious.

Two points need to be emphasized therefore in considering the development of co-operation in humans ; first that it is a natural process like growth, and will proceed spontaneously in a good environment; and secondly, that it can only develop satisfactorily when conditions are favourable. Anything which leads to distrust and fear of others will interfere with its progress.

But whilst co-operation is undoubtedly natural to children it cannot be said to be their only social activity. Like primitive men who also co-operate in simple ways children fight.

Now no one needs to be told that children fight, yet it is interesting to have detailed observations of the situations which provoke their fights and of the children's motives in ' going to war '. These situations can be described under two heads :

(1) Situations which threaten the loss of possessions or affection.

(2) Situations of failure or anxiety over the accomplishment of a task.

(1) *Situations which threaten the loss of possessions or affection.* There is hardly anything which a child likes of which he does not want exclusive possession and for which he is not prepared, if necessary, to fight. The very small child cannot tolerate either sharing or taking turns for he is unable to trust any one with the objects of his desire. These objects are of many kinds. It is not only his toys and clothes and other little things which he likes ; possessiveness may spread also to abstract articles such as nursery rhymes and tunes, and a child may become angry with another for wearing her favourite colour.

' Harold and Paul felt a keen sense of property in the nursery rhymes and songs they had heard at home, or in gramophone records of a kind they had there. No one else had the right to sing or hear these things without their permission. All the children felt that anything was " theirs " if they had used it first, or had made it, even with material that itself belonged to all. Duncan and others felt a thing was " theirs " if they had " thought " of it, or " mentioned for it first," and so on.'[1]

Another important observation of Isaacs is that ' neither the pleasure of ownership nor the chagrin of envy bears much relation to the intrinsic value of the things owned or coveted '. It is enough for another child to want a thing for that thing to be valuable, indeed essential. Many instances are described of one child wanting the unused possession of another, only to awaken an immediate desire for the thing in the owner.

' While Dan (3.8) was occupied with something else, he saw Harold (5.0) take one of his engine books, which he had left on the shelf, to read. Harold put it down on the table and remarked that he was going to read it " all the morning." Dan immediately said : " *I* want it," and tried to take it from Harold, and screamed and cried. He took it away in the end.'[2]

' Lena (3.9) always wants to have any object which another child happens to be enjoying, e.g. the tricycle or engine, and tries to get it forcibly.'[3]

[1] Op. cit., p. 222.
[2] The figures in brackets refer to the children's ages in years and months at the time of the event quoted.
[3] Op. cit., pp. 35 and 39.

But perhaps the most important objects of which a child wants possession are the people who afford him pleasure and whom he loves. In this respect children are very like the apes who, as Zuckermann says, treat females fundamentally as material objects. Isaacs notes that aggressive behaviour from the motive of rivalry for the possession of a person was both more frequent and gave rise to more acute tension of feeling than did rivalry over material possessions.

' George (4.5), seeing Miss B. sit down to the table with bricks, left his modelling and went at once to sit beside her. Dan (3.8) and Frank (5.3) also went and a squabble ensued as to who should sit next to Miss B. As none of them was willing to give way, Miss B. got up and went back to the modelling table. Dan did not notice this and went on building, but George and Frank saw it at once and left the bricks, and went back to the modelling table to sit one each side of her. When, presently, Dan realized what had happened he came again and cried and screamed to sit beside her.'[1]

Anyone who has looked after children will recognize these instances as absolutely typical of childhood. The intensity of hatred engendered is terrific.

Rivalry is particularly noticeable when a new child enters a group. ' The hostile reaction of a group of young children to new-comers . . . seems to me quite undiscriminating . . . it may be felt and expressed even before the child has actually appeared, on mere hearing that he is to come.' One child expressed this assumption by remarking that people ' don't like you—because they have not seen you before.'[2] The new-comer is called silly, exception is taken to the way he dresses or to the way he walks. Such hostility is clearly the expression of a fear that he will be a rival for toys and for the love and admiration of the grown-ups. The new-comer is felt to be a menace and it is not until he has been in the group for a time that the others become reassured and he is tolerated. It is consequently not surprising that the new-comers themselves adopt an attitude of fear or hostility. ' An attitude of hostility to all the other children seems to be the primary active response of any young child on entering a group.'

A special example of a new-comer arousing intense feelings of jealousy and hostility is when a new baby is born and an

---

[1] Op. cit., p. 50.   [2] Op. cit., p. 255.

older child has to take a back place. Hatred of the new baby
may be mixed with pleasure and affection and much depends
upon the way the situation is handled, but probably no child
up to the age of about six years can tolerate what it feels to
be a rejection from its mother without at times hating and
wanting to annihilate the rival. It is true that some mothers
so much prefer their first child that it is the baby who becomes
the jealous one. But the usual sequence to a birth is that the
elder child feels cast out and resentful, although if the jealousy
is dealt with sympathetically it will gradually disappear.

Of course, sometimes the hatred remains concealed. When
parents and nurses add insult to injury by being angry with
the resentful outcast, he is likely to make an effort to appear
to like the new-comer. But often there is no concealment.
Many are the occasions when an older child is found attacking
the younger with a nursery weapon. For instance, a little
girl of four was caught in the act of hitting her younger sister
aged one with the lid of the Noah's Ark. Again and again
mothers of difficult children complain that their chief trouble
is the way the child maltreats the younger ones. On investigation it is usually found that most of the difficulties arose soon
after the birth of the younger child and that jealousy was
acute and unsympathetically handled.

A worried mother writes :

'But it is his attitude to his little sister that worries me
most. I cannot make him remember he is older or instil the
smallest bit of the protective attitude into him. He wants
to be treated exactly as she is and to have everything she
has, and takes anything from her, often hitting her or
knocking her over until I am really scared to leave them
together. I may say she sticks up for herself well, but there
is three and a half years' difference. When talked to he is
all affection and promises at once never to do it again, but
not five minutes elapse before he is as bad as ever.'[1]

Even in children who, on the whole, are well disposed
towards their younger brothers or sisters, hostility may usually
be detected. For instance, Isaacs reports the case of a little
girl of four who had been sensibly treated and who welcomed
the new baby : ' She's only sweet ! She's just what I wanted ! '
Yet when the baby was six months old she had ' A nasty
dream.' ' Nurse came in with R. and I hit her on the head
. . . and then there was something very nasty ! I *can't* tell

you that. . . .' A month or two later she punched her mother and was generally tiresome when her mother was feeding the baby and when the time came for the baby's cot to be moved into her room, again became very resentful.[1]

The overwhelming importance of the possession of the mother (or mother substitute) is exemplified again when another adult appears and wants to talk to her. Very small children show undisguised hostility in such a situation, attempting to part the grown-ups, becoming fractious and so on. The constant tendency for little children to become more difficult when two or more grown-ups are present than when with one alone is well known. The child is happy with its nurse and becomes difficult when mother appears or vice versa. This usually leads to the nurse concluding with satisfaction that the mother is bad for the child and the mother feeling that the child prefers her to the nurse.[2]

'The degree of Frank's sensitiveness to the presence of adult rivals was most · striking. Whenever Dan's father entered the school, for instance, Frank (5 to 6) changed in a moment from active gaiety to sulky destructiveness. Penelope (3 to 4), too, seemed rarely able to be loving both to a man friend and a woman friend at the same time. Nor did Dan (3 to 4), throughout the first year of the school, find himself able to love both Mrs. I. and her assistant at once.'[3]

These rivalries and the hatred springing from them will be further discussed in the next section. For the moment we may conclude that one of the chief sources of hatred and aggression in childhood are situations in which there is deprivation or threatened deprivation. Any frustration of the desire to possess toys or food or the love and approval of others leads to outbursts of anger and aggression. Isaacs remarks that the anger is often quite as intense as if life itself was threatened. The actual threat, of course, is to the sources of

---

[1] Op. cit., pp. 196–200.

[2] Cf. Isaacs. 'In my notes of recent years, I have gathered a great many instances of the way in which children who are friendly and amenable when with one grown-up only will become fractious and perverse as soon as another enters on the scene. A child may be happy and obedient with either the mother or the father, but disagreeable when both are there. He may contentedly obey the nurse when she has him alone, and be difficult when the mother comes into the nursery. He may be good with either mother or nurse separately, and contrary with the two together. It seems indeed a universal tendency of little children to become more difficult when two or more grown-ups are present than when with one alone.'

[3] Op. cit., p. 237.

what make life worth while—the sources of pleasure and satisfaction. Toys and nursery rhymes give pleasure and must, therefore, be retained at all costs. People are also sources of pleasure, both because they give food and toys and also because they give affection and care. They must, therefore, be kept well-disposed and any rival for their attentions beaten off.

(2) *Situations of anxiety and failure over the accomplishment of a task.* It is not difficult to understand the aggression which springs from motives of possessiveness. Desires for material objects and for affection, and an outbreak of anger when these desires are thwarted by others are such commonplace events as ordinarily to be taken for granted.

The origins of aggression to be discussed under this heading, however, are far less easily appreciated and their importance commonly greatly underestimated. The possession of material objects and of the affection of friends depends as much upon our own activities as upon those of others. Affection may be lost through our own bad behaviour as well as through the competitive behaviour of others. Material objects can be lost or broken by ourselves as well as being stolen. Observation shows that bad-temper in children is just as frequently due to *self-frustration* as it is to the more obvious frustration by others.

' Moreover, the element of rivalry in this moody hostility was with certain of the children very clearly bound up with a general sense of their own relative helplessness or ineffectiveness. Cecil was a particularly clear example of this. He was a large but loose-jointed and clumsy child, who could do nothing skilfully. Everything he tried to build fell down, to his own distress and chagrin. He could not even wash his own hands when he first came to school at four years of age, having been trained to no sort of independence at home. It was very noticeable how his aggressiveness became less as his skill and self-confidence grew greater.'[1]

The mother of another child wrote as follows :

' She is an only child (3.6), fully developed, of normal and regular habits. The trouble at present is that she takes fits of crying without any obvious reason, accompanied by stamping of feet, and very often disobedience at these times. . . . She was playing in the garden with her doll's pram, while I was cutting the grass—suddenly she started crying—on being questioned as to what was wrong—had she

[1] Op. cit., p. 245.

fallen, or had anything frightened her—she refused to answer and continued to cry and scream for about an hour. Sometime later on being questioned as to what was wrong, she told me she could not manage her pram on to the lawn. I tried to explain to her, that if only she had asked I would have helped her—but she evaded my reasoning.'[1]

In both these instances the bad temper clearly resulted from a sense of frustration, but in neither was it another person who was to blame.

If children can get into tempers about such comparatively trivial failures as an inability to build brick castles or push a pram on to the lawn, it is not surprising that an inability to earn the approval and affection of the grown-ups should cause even greater consternation. Thus it comes about that some of the worst outbursts of anger in childhood occur when a child is told that it is naughty or even when it only anticipates disapproval from the grown-ups.

'Benjie (4.1), after lunch, dropped the water-jug accidentally. He looked quickly at Mrs. I., laughed excitedly, then kicked it across the room ; he was about to kick it downstairs. Mrs. I. asked him not to do so, but before she could get near he had done so, and broken it. Then he was very defiant, shouting : " I'll hit you in the face ; I'll not come to school any more," and so on. This was clearly remorse that took the form of defiance.

'When Benjie spat into the pudding dish, and Mrs. I hastily said : " Now you can't have any pudding," he threw his plate on the floor and broke it. Then he cried very bitterly in anger and defiance.'[2]

In both these cases Benjie became aggressive as a result of doing something which he feared had earned him Mrs. Isaacs' displeasure. Probably in each case he expected punishment and part of his aggression was to combat that, but other evidence suggests that the anger is partly at least directed against himself as the result of *self-dissatisfaction*.

For instance, a boy of fourteen had always suffered from severe outbursts of temper. These had usually been put down to 'naughtiness.' Observation, however, showed that they occurred whenever he made a mistake and failed in some way. One day on his way to school he found he had forgotten his season ticket. He at once flew into a rage with the ticket-

[1] Op. cit., pp. 70–71.   [2] Op. cit., p. 172.

collector who refused to allow him to pass. On returning home he became abusive to his mother and hit his little brother.

Episodes such as this are frequent in anyone's life. Missing an easy shot, arriving at the station to see the train just going out, upsetting the coffee over one's hostess' gown, breaking a favourite bowl, these are the incidents which put us out of temper with ourselves and in a bad temper with everyone else. What is so particularly mortifying about them is that we have only ourselves to blame and that we cannot legitimately vent our wrath on others. The difficulties of such situations will be discussed at length in the next section and are held by the authors to be of great importance in understanding aggressive behaviour.

In addition to the frustration and anger resulting from the actions either of other people or ourselves, anger may arise from impersonal events. For instance, the picnic we have planned for a hot summer's day may be washed out by a thunderstorm or a motor trip spoiled by a puncture. In neither case is it anyone's fault—the material world is to blame. Without further study it is difficult to estimate the relative importance of such events in causing anger, but there can be no doubt that such happenings make children and grown-ups bad-tempered.

Incidentally, as will be described later, these impersonal frustrations are rarely if ever *felt* as impersonal. Probably because most of the child's early frustrations come from people, children assume that even natural events like rain or cold are the outcome of some personal action. Their anger is consequently diverted against the supposed culprit. This tendency to inculpate and to vent wrath on someone who has had nothing to do with the incident provoking it has been constantly emphasised by psycho-analysts, and appear to us to be of fundamental importance in understanding the origins of war.

Before considering the psycho-analytic evidence regarding hatred and aggression in detail, one further characteristic of aggression in childhood which is easily observed requires special emphasis. This is its violence. Children are notoriously unkind to one another. Of course they are often very kind as well, but we have only to remember the fights and teasing and bullying which go on in any nursery or school, even the best regulated, to realize that children, like baboons, are not natural pacifists. Descriptions such as these from worried mothers remind us how violent and merciless children can be.

'I must write and tell you of my experience with this "jealous hostility." I took your advice and a month ago two little two-year-olds came to live with us as companions for my son of the same age. They looked so sweet together— all red-cheeked, curly-haired, adored only children, but, unfortunately, *they hated each other*. I was in despair. I'd no idea babies could be so horrid to each other. We daren't leave them alone for a moment—such shrieks and yells would come from the nursery. They would pull each other's hair out by the handful—scratch, bite, push each other down—tread on each other. It was heart-breaking. I've seen chickens persecuting a lame fowl—almost pecking it to death. These babies were just little animals. If one fell and cried because of the bump, the other two rushed over to pull his hair and increase the yells. " Pip " loved to bang the others on the head with a brick.'

Another writes :

' My other difficulty is about the unkindness of the two elder ones (girl aged 6.6 and boy aged 5.6) to the child of three and a half. They have always resented her existence, I know, though I tried to avoid making them jealous. They are devoted to each other and are quite kind to the baby, but Cecilia's life is really hardly worth living because they are so nasty to her. They tease her constantly by running off with her doll's blankets or knocking over her tea-cups or just by pushing her away (she is learning to tease, too), and also in more subtle ways by making her say foolish things and then jeering at her. She, poor thing, never remembers how she's been caught before, and constantly gets caught again, and she is old enough now to mind considerably.'[1]

Even the desire to kill others is not alien to the childish mind. It was a comparatively normal if aggressive small boy who, on being told by his father that *his* father was dead, earnestly enquired : " Did you kill him and stamp on him ? " Such comments are typical of children who are allowed to express their feelings freely.

' Jessica (3.5) accidentally tore a card which had been sent by Miss C. to all the children. Dan (4.9) said he would " get a policeman to put her in prison," and " I'll kill her, because I hate her." '
' Dan (5.0) spoke of the tricycle which Tommy (4.1) had

<hr />

[1] Op. cit., pp. 59–60.

lent him. Dan said : " Tommy lent it to me while he
was ill—I wish he was dead, then I could have it always ! " [1]

It can therefore be taken as established that bitter hatreds
are inseparable from childhood, but this does not mean that
they cannot vary enormously in degree. Much can be done
by sympathetic and tolerant handling of children, and it is
interesting to find that of Mrs. Isaacs' group the more crudely
aggressive were those who were whipped at home. Although
so far as we know no definite research has been done on this
queston, it is the impression of most people who work with
children that violence begets violence and that little good and
much harm comes from attempts to beat children into pacific
behaviour.

Conclusions.

The main facts which have been established by the modern
studies of aggression in childhood can now be summarized.

(1) The situations which provoke outbursts of aggression
are of two types. Any threat to valued possessions such as
toys, food, the affections of others and of course life itself
constitutes one type. Within this are numerous acute
situations of jealousy and rivalry such as the birth of a new
baby into a family or the entry of a new child into a school.
In these situations other people, adults or children, cause the
frustration and become the objects of hatred. The other
type, which is less generally recognized, consists of situations
in which the child frustrates himself by his own incapacities or
wilfulness. He alone is to blame if he inadvertently knocks
over his brick castle or earns disapproval by tiresome behaviour.
In such cases the object of hatred is not an external person
but the child himself.

(2) Aggression in childhood is conspicuous for its violence.
The desire to kill a rival is often freely expressed and sometimes,
especially in early childhood, attempted. Numerous cases of
children of three to five hitting and hurting their younger
brothers or sisters are instanced.

(3) Although all children have violent propensities their
violence is of varying degrees and depends upon the way they
are treated. It is common experience that the most violent
are those who have themselves been subjected to violence.
This belief together with much else connected with aggression
in childhood lends itself to accurate research which we hope
soon to see undertaken.

[1] Op. cit., p. 38.

(3) PSYCHO-ANALYTIC STUDIES OF AGGRESSION

Aggression in apes and children is relatively easily studied by the simple method of observing the animals in a group. This is more difficult to carry out with adult humans and so far as we know has never been attempted. But there does exist a different body of data regarding the aggressive feelings and acts of civilized man which we believe to be extremely relevant to the problem of war. This is the data collected by psycho-analysts in the course of their therapeutic work.[1]

Experience has shown that all patients who suffer from neurotic or psychotic symptoms show abnormalities in the development of their aggressive feelings. Some are bitter, angry people who are constantly complaining that other people are unkind or morally bad, others are quiet and sensitive souls who are afraid to stand up for themselves and will eat any amount of humble pie in order to avoid a row. Hatred in the one case seems to be over-developed and in the other either atrophied or exaggeratedly controlled. And not only are mental sufferers abnormal in these ways, but further work has demonstrated that many of their symptoms are the direct result of their aggressive impulses being either faultily developed or controlled. As a consequence an intensive study of the aggressive propensities of all types of patients has been forced upon psycho-analysts.

This work has very largely extended our knowledge of aggression in man. It has revealed the ubiquity of hatred, its presence where formerly it was unsuspected and its frequent irrationality. People who normally pass for peaceful loving individuals have sometimes been found to be eaten up by jealousy and hatred, whilst those who appear always in a bad temper with friends and relatives have been found to be

---

[1] Apart from certain speculative theories, such as that of the Death Instinct, psycho-analytic theory has been evolved from a close examination of the feelings, thoughts (including phantasies and dreams) and behaviour of patients in a certain controlled relationship with the physician. The scientific validity of such conclusions is sometimes questioned. Whilst admitting that it is far from a perfect scientific procedure, the authors hold that its results if interpreted cautiously are reliable. Many of the more important observations have been repeated in the less formal setting of the nursery and much of the material quoted here is of such a kind. Although the check of controlled experiment is as yet impossible, theories can be tested for their ability to promote accurate prediction. The objection that the material of observation is abnormal carries little weight. Not only have many people who commonly pass for normal been analysed, but in other branches of science breakdowns of the normal are regarded as specially illuminating. The debt of physiology to pathology is enormous, whilst physics nowadays is largely concerned with the examination of phenomena which never occur in Nature outside the laboratory.

prompted by feelings of self-dissatisfaction and self-hatred more often than by any realistic external frustration. Psychoanalysts have consequently been compelled to take a very different view of the hatred and aggression even of normal man from that which is commonly held. Because of the limited space available no attempt has been made to discuss all the relevant issues in this section. Instead we have preferred to concentrate attention on a few of the most important conclusions, giving examples of the evidence upon which they are founded.

One of the earliest and most fundamental of psycho-analytic discoveries was that people could do hostile things without being aware either of feelings of hatred or of the nature of their act. This led to the theory of ' unconscious hatred,'[1] which states that people can be motivated by feelings of hatred of which they are not conscious and actuated by hostile impulses of whose existence they have no knowledge. This notion of people being influenced by motives of which they are unconscious is one which still meets with much theoretical opposition. Yet the empirical evidence is quite unequivocal. For instance a physician was called out urgently to a case and had to wire to postpone the appointment of another patient. This other patient was of the excessively polite type who always found it exceedingly difficult to experience any feelings of antagonism within himself. It was, therefore, completely in character for him to take the postponement in an apparently philosophical mood and agree readily to the later appointment. Yet when he came, on preceding the doctor into his consulting-room, he shut the door in the doctor's face. This man had been aware of no feelings of resentment at the postponement of his appointment and was equally unaware of what he had done. Yet a discussion showed that slamming the door had been no accident—that it was in fact prompted by feelings of resentment which had been repressed. For the postponement had caused him a good deal of inconvenience, and on receiving it he had said to himself : ' I must be careful to write a very polite letter—I must not let any feelings of irritation get expressed in it.'

---

[1] It is probably more accurate to speak of ' unconscious aggressive impulses.' It is often objected that *feelings* cannot be unconscious and that, since hatred is a feeling, hatred cannot be unconscious. There can be no such terminological objection to the concept of unconscious *impulses* influencing our actions. Many of the things we do, breathing or walking for instance, are obviously unconsciously motivated and there is no *a priori* reason to doubt that aggressive impulses can remain unconscious also. Nevertheless the slightly inaccurate term ' unconscious hatred ' is expressive and useful.

Freud has collected numerous similar instances in which people's real feelings influence their actions without their being aware of what is happening.[1] He quotes the case of a young man who lost a pencil to which he was much attached, a loss which he regarded as an unfortunate accident. Investigation showed that a few days previously he had received a very critical letter from his brother-in-law and that this brother-in-law had presented him with the pencil. The loss was clearly no accident but an expression of resentment with his critical brother-in-law.

The breaking of crockery by domestics is another instance of purposeful accidents. Plates ' come to pieces in my hands ' far more frequently after the maid has been reprimanded than when she has been praised. Indeed it is impossible to criticize some maids without paying for it in breakages.

Examples could easily be multiplied. Misprints and slips of the tongue frequently express the true feelings of hostility which it was intended should be hidden. For instance, in a war correspondent's account of meeting a famous general whose infirmities were pretty well known, a reference to the general was printed as ' this battle-scared veteran.' Next day an apology appeared which read ' the words of course should have been " this bottle-scarred veteran." '[2]

Most grown-ups dislike to feel that they have been prompted in their action by hostile or other repressed impulses and are inclined to call such episodes accidents. In this respect children are perhaps more honest. For them there is the convention of ' by mistake on purpose '. The hostile feelings are there admitted and only partially disowned. As they grow older, however, the ' on purpose ' gets omitted and the action is believed to be purely ' by mistake.' In this people may be quite honest. In the case of the man who shut the door in the doctor's face there was no doubt that he was quite unaware of his feelings of anger and revenge for being locked out himself, and quite unaware that the apparent accident had been impelled by a deliberate purpose. Although the significance of the incident was fairly readily recognized when it was pointed out to him, there are of course many people who would completely repudiate any suggestion that they had been influenced by such feelings. There seems, in fact, to be every degree of awareness and unawareness of real motives. We may know our feelings and deliberately act upon them. We may know our feelings and partially repudiate them, yet permit

[1] Freud, *Introductory Lectures on Psycho-Analysis.*
[2] Quoted by Freud, op. cit.

them some expression, or we may repudiate them altogether. In this latter case the result is often that a hostile action is carried out without the person's conscious choice or intention, and sometimes without his even knowing what he has done.

Clearly the existence of these unconscious hostile impulses is important, especially as psycho-analysts have discovered them in greater or less degree in every patient who has been treated.[1] If individuals can be actuated by unconscious hatred in their private lives, it seems not unreasonable to suppose that they may be so motivated in affairs of State. But for the moment we will confine ourselves to the individual and the problem as to why certain impulses are disowned or *repressed*.

Psycho-analysis has been deeply concerned with this problem of repression, for the good reason that the radical cure of neurotics is impossible so long as active impulses remain unconscious. In investigating this problem Freud soon discovered that the repression of impulses was no accidental condition, but the result of the purposeful action of powerful mental forces. Patients refused to admit that they were motivated by jealousy or rage—for some reason they *could* not become aware of such feelings, though they might be obvious to an external observer from their every word and action.

The next question for solution was therefore the nature of the repressing forces. It was soon obvious that they were associated with conscience and the sense of shame, that repression in fact was a more drastic form of the common experience of wanting to forget something of which one feels ashamed. But conscience on investigation proves to be no simple thing and psycho-analysts have been forced to postulate a more extensive psychic agency which includes the conscious conscience and other forces as well. This has been termed the super-ego.

It is impossible here to enter in detail into the controversial theory of the origins of the super-ego. It is sufficient to say that all psycho-analysts are agreed that there exists in the mind a combination of forces which are represented in consciousness by conscience and which are responsible for many feelings and impulses being banished from a person's awareness of themselves. Of these repressed impulses the sexual and the aggressive are the most important, although there is no impulse which is not liable to repression. Since, however, we

---

[1] In this psycho-analysts have been preceded by Eastern mystics who have apparently long recognized the ubiquity of 'latent hatred.' Psycho-analysts are the first to have studied it scientifically, however.

are chiefly concerned here with the repression of aggression these other impulses will not often be referred to.

In the growth of the repressing agency two main forces seem to be operative :

(1) The most obvious is the external pressure which parents and other adults bring to bear upon children through disapproval and punishment. Of course punishments can be of various kinds and it is not always the crudest which are the most cruel and repressive. Thrashings seem to produce hating and rebellious children as often as they make them meek and obedient. On the other hand in skilled hands threats such as ' I'll never love you any more,' or, ' You'll be sent away to a home,' or even a pained nod of the head will curb all but the most defiant of children. (Of course, it is rarely realized that threats of this kind are fully as cruel as the most savage thrashings.)

The effect of these measures will naturally be to make the child attempt to hide its real feelings. If a child is sufficiently often scolded or punished for showing displeasure or resentment, these feelings will be disguised. As time goes on the child may even succeed in hiding them from itself and finally perhaps cease altogether to be aware of their existence. But this process does not necessarily exterminate the impulses which may continue to influence conduct without the person being aware of the fact.

Yet another mode of stamping out hatred in children is to appeal to their pity and love. This is an exploitation of the second major force.

(2) Quite apart from external forces which may be brought to bear on a child to curb his natural impulses is a purely subjective process which is often greatly underestimated. This is the child's feelings of affection for its parents and the inevitable repulsion it has for its own feelings of anger for them. As was emphasized in the last chapter, children are as naturally co-operative and sociable as they are selfish and anti-social. They have spontaneous feelings of love and concern for their relatives as well as feelings of jealousy and hatred for them. This is shown very dramatically when a child after getting into a furious temper with its mother becomes miserable and penitent and extremely solicitous for her welfare.[1] Mothers frequently fail to take these protestations seriously, but experience shows that in the vast majority of cases they are to be taken with the utmost seriousness. For

[1] See case quoted on p. 98.

after being in a temper children feel terrified not only of
losing their parents' love, but also lest they should have
actually harmed their parents.   For they realize, more or less
consciously, that when they are in a temper the people whom
they love most stand in real danger.   An attempt to banish
these dangerous hostile feelings not unnaturally follows.

Of course it is always difficult to know to what extent the
moral views of children have been influenced by upbringing,
but observations have shown that it is not only children who
have been brought up in a moralizing atmosphere who develop
an abhorrence of the ' naughty,' both in themselves and in
others.   Like hope, the idea of naughtiness seems to spring
eternal in the human breast.   Attempts may be made to
minimize it by avoiding blaming children, but the very fact
that children are inclined to actions which the most tolerant
grown-up cannot like inevitably breeds the feeling.   For
apart from any moral laws or principles, children come to
feel as naughty anything which the grown-ups do not like.
This is typified by the following incidents.

> ' Alfred (4.2) and Herbert (2.11) were watching the mice,
> and making them run up and down the stairs in the mouse-
> box.   When they couldn't make them do this, they called
> them " naughty mice "—" Aren't they naughty mice ? "
> Mrs. I. said :   " Are they ? " and they replied :   " They
> won't do what we want, so aren't they *naughty* ? " '
> ' Dan (4.1) was on the river with his father, and defecated
> in his trousers.   He burst into deep sobs of distress, and
> said :   " Oh, what shall I do ! oh, Daddy, *Daddy*."   Dan
> had never been scolded or even slightly reproached for such
> " accidents " which were very rare.'
> ' Dan gave Harold a motor bus.   Harold (5.2) put it in
> the cloakroom, and when his mother came, she said it was
> not convenient to take it home that day.   Harold was
> very angry at this, and hit his mother several times and
> said hostile things.   She said she was very sorry, but she
> could not do it.   The next day she told Mrs. I. how, all
> the way home, he kept hitting her and saying hostile things,
> and how a long time afterwards he asked her :   " Do you
> still love me ? " and when she said " Yes," he said :   " What,
> after all that ? " '[1]

Hostility, destructiveness, dirtiness, and greed, all strongly
developed in children, will almost always be regarded as

[1] Op. cit., pp. 182, 179 and 178.

naughty, although details will be much influenced by the attitude of mother and nurse.

This subjective source of guilt carrying with it a need to repress hostile impulses is more difficult for the majority of people to understand than is the external source. It is consequently worth while dealing with it more fully. Its origin lies in the inclination of human beings to feel both hate and love for the same person. This propensity, known technically as *ambivalence*, is of the greatest importance for the understanding not only of repression but of the whole problem of hate and aggression in man.

Intensive investigation of the motives and feelings of children and adults has revealed a far greater complexity of emotional attitude than is usually recognized. The common man says that he likes X and hates Y and believes this to be true. But careful observation of his moods, thoughts, phantasies and dreams show that his love for X is not so pure as he thought, that feelings of hatred enter in, whilst his outspoken hatred for Y is partly manufactured to avoid envy and may conceal admiration and love. This relationship in which a person alternates between feelings of love and hatred for another is, of course, particularly characteristic of childhood. At one moment a child is happy and affectionate towards his mother, at the next in a towering rage with her for refusing him some trifle. After a short while the incident is forgotten and feelings of love restored. All children pass through such stages, indeed it is taken for granted. What is not so commonly recognized is that similar alternations are extremely frequent also in adults. They are especially noticeable in a patient's personal attitude to the analyst. For instance, a girl of twenty who was being treated wrote a note to her physician one day saying that she was sorry she was unable to come as she had a cold, adding almost effusive thanks for the improvement which treatment had made in her condition. Yet when next she came she was in a very bad temper, saying that she was as bad as she had ever been, that she had had awful thoughts of hurting people and great depression. On investigation it turned out that she had hoped and expected a note from her analyst in reply and that all this bad temper had come on when she realized that she would not get one. She remembered often getting into similar rages with her mother when she was a child and feeling dreadful afterwards for having thought such unkind things about her. It was clear in this case that at the age of twenty she was behaving towards the analyst exactly as she had towards her mother when she was five or less.

Such episodes are absolutely typical. It is true that they are more frequent and more intense the more neurotic the patient, but there are few people who do not exhibit such alternations sometimes. And not only can impulses of love and hate for the same person alternate with one another, but experience has shown that they may actually be operative at one and the same moment and result in thoughts and acts which partake of each.

The attack by MacMahon upon King Edward VIII is a good example. It was clear from the evidence that he was actuated both by a desire to kill the King and also by a desire to protect him. One of his stories was that, having received news that an attempt was to be made upon the King's life, he phoned the police to warn them. Obviously the threat came in fact from himself and it was against himself that he was warning the police. During the procession he seems to have been in a state of great agitation. Finally, when the King came by, his action was a perfect compromise between attacking and protecting him. He attacked the King by throwing his revolver at him. This whilst serious in form was negligible in results and, moreover, had the desirable effect of having the attacker taken into custody.

That this is not a fanciful reconstruction of the episode is shown by the statement of the man who murdered President Doumer of France. He described how he felt impelled to shoot the President on a certain day, but yet did his best to prevent himself doing so. First he got drunk in a café, then gave himself up to a policeman, telling him that he was going to shoot the President and that he had better be arrested first. Unfortunately the policeman had a sense of humour and was indulgent with the drunkard, with the result that the President was assassinated.

In these instances the process of repression is obviously breaking down ; the murderous impulses are getting out of control and inadvertently venting themselves upon people different from the originals. (We may surmise that in each case there had been displacement of hatred from the original object, probably the father, on to the titular head of the State.) More commonly the person who suffers from these conflicting impulses is completely ignorant of one of them, usually the hostility, and believes himself actuated only by love.

These psycho-analytic observations of neurotics are amply confirmed by common experience of normal people. The woman who protests undying love for her husband, yet nags him continually and is jealous of his work and men friends, the man who loves his children, yet beats them unmercifully when they are troublesome or make a noise are well known. And after all it is not surprising that the people who mean most to us should have power to evoke most feelings of anger. For, as observations on children and monkeys demonstrate, aggression is aroused when desires are frustrated. The stronger the desire, therefore, the more likely the frustration and the fiercer the aggression. Many instances can be given of situations where bitter hatred is called forth for a person who is otherwise loved, because he or she frustrates. A man will feel angry with a girl who leaves him for another man. A woman will feel angry with her husband for not earning more money or not providing her with a child.

The ambivalence of childhood has already been commented upon but needs especial emphasis because it is during childhood that passions are at their height and the repressing forces of the super-ego first develop. We have only to watch a group of children playing to witness the rapidity with which friendships dissolve and hatreds appear, enmities are reconciled and alliances formed. But in addition to the obvious occasions when a child is inspired to hatred for the parents or playmates whom it usually loves there are several situations which call for greater description because of the intensity of emotion and conflict generated.

One such is when a mother denies her baby the breast when it wants it. Instead of the affection inseparable from enjoyed satisfaction the baby screams and kicks in a paroxysm of rage and anger. Instead of loving its mother, it hates her. Since this is the first personal relationship which a child knows it is hardly surprising to discover that it often influences later relations very deeply.

Another occasion when love and hatred are mixed is when a child sees its mother with a new baby. Examples have already been given of children who are bitterly jealous of the new baby, a jealousy which engenders great hatred both for the rival and for the traitor mother. Yet the child may usually be most devoted to its mother and at times welcome the new baby as an object of love : ' It is just what I wanted ! '

Still another is the jealousy aroused by the sight of the two parents being together. A child may be very fond of his father, yet jealous and resentful when he interrupts his play with his mother. This is obviously a very special case of the rivalry and anger which children feel when any two adults are together.

For instance, an only boy of five was always very upset if

his parents went out alone, leaving him at home with the maid.
His jealousy was particularly noticeable on Sunday morning
when his parents slept later. He used to knock on his parents'
door and want to come in. When he found that they refused
him admittance until later, he hit on the dodge of preparing
their early-morning tea for them. This gained him admittance.
His father who had no knowledge of psychology realized that
his son regarded him as a rival for his mother's love.

Moreover this rivalry is not undiscriminating. A sexual
motive enters in. Freud has been severely criticized for
drawing attention to the sexual preferences of young children,
but it is really a matter of common nursery experience. Little
boys take more interest in women, little girls in men.

> ' Penelope (3.6) came to tea with Mrs. I. There were
> several women there, all friendly and sympathetic to children.
> But Penelope gave all her interest to the one man present,
> making him play various games with her, caressing him and
> sitting on his knee, monopolizing his attention all the time
> and not readily allowing him to take any notice of any one
> else.'[1]

In view of these observations, it is not surprising to discover
that acute feelings of jealousy are constantly aroused in children
by the affectionate relation of their two parents. For there is
both the jealousy of the two adults being together, which the
child feels to be a threat to his possession of either, and also
the jealousy of sexual preference. The ambivalent feelings
thereby aroused cause great conflict and have been termed the
Œdipus complex by Freud. Psycho-analytic literature is full
of examples of it.

In each of these instances hatred is aroused for the very
person who is also most loved. The child welcomes the new
baby, yet hates it for usurping his position. He loves his
mother, yet hates her for giving more time and affection to the
new-comer than to himself. He loves and admires his father,
yet wishes him dead on the occasions when he steals his mother
from him. Such ambivalent relationships are quite inseparable
from childhood and begin when the infant in arms first screams
with rage at his mother for not feeding him on demand.

Now it may be said that much of this is so obvious as to
be of no importance. It is true that Freud did not discover
the existence of ambivalence any more than Newton was the
first to observe apples fall from trees. Freud's claim to fame

[1] Isaacs, op. cit., p. 51.

lies in his recognition of the universality of ambivalence in human relations and of the torturing conflicts to which it gives rise. For experience shows that, as a person develops, an ambivalent relationship becomes more and more intolerable.

In the first place there is the fear of retaliatory punishment which is seen in children of two or three. But apart from the possibility of punishment, ambivalence obviously interferes with the permanent friendly relation with adults which children so much desire. Moreover, as has already been remarked, it begets remorse ; for no one can get into a rage to the point of desiring to kill someone whom they are fond of without subsequently feeling regret and shame. Promptings from moralizing adults will no doubt increase them, but all the evidence suggests that their birth is spontaneous, arising inevitably from the conflict of ambivalence. The following conversation between two three-year-olds gives an illustration of its beginnings.

' Tommy and Martin were in the sand-pit, and talked to each other thus : Martin : " Do you love me ? " " Yes, I love you." Martin : " I love you—I'm not going to hit you again. Shall I hit you again ? No, I'm not going to hit you again." Martin repeated this two or three times.'[1]

The conflict is clearly expressed. On the one hand the child does not want to give up the luxury of expressing his aggression. On the other he does not want to interrupt his friendship nor suffer remorse from hurting his friend. It is an awkward dilemma, solved in this case apparently by Martin deciding to control his desire to hit Tommy. Unfortunately the solution is often less philosophically arrived at. A scolding adult demanding peace or the victim being seriously hurt might easily have upset the achievement of voluntary control and resulted in a wholesale repression of the desire to hit.

The difference between conscious control and unconscious repression is no doubt one of degree, but the result is profoundly different. For in the one case the person remains master in his own house, in the other the impulse is banished and control therefore impossible. It is the difference between socializing a dangerous criminal whilst maintaining supervision over him and banishing him to another land where he may, for all we know, continue to plot against us. So long as we retain responsibility for our impulses, as with our criminals, we stand in no danger from them. The problem arises when

---

[1] Isaacs, op. cit., p. 277.

impulses are banished and the person succeeds in attaining gnorance of his own wishes. These wishes may then influence hs actions without his realizing it and give rise to the various unconscious hostile acts which have already bnee illustrated.

The formation of the super-ego and the repression of anti-social impulses is, as we have seen, largely the result of the existence of ambivalence. It is in order to avoid the conflicts inseparable from an ambivalent relation that repression is undertaken and anti-social impulses such as aggression and greed stamped down. The result of this simple repression is commonly the non-aggressive, over-polite, over-conscientious type of person, who may none the less be responsible unintentionally for much unkindness. A knowledge of the existence of ambivalent feelings and of the mechanism of repression as a way of dealing with them is obviously of great importance for an understanding of human social relations.

But there are other methods of solving the conflict of ambivalence in addition to repression which are perhaps of even greater social importance. For some of them lead to the expression of violent hatred and aggression upon quite inappropriate people, people who have had nothing whatever to do with the stimulation of such feelings. Psycho-analysts have discovered that anger and aggression are constantly directed away from original objects on to other and often completely irrational ones, and it is because of this that they have approached the problem of war sceptical of rational explanations. For if individuals may hate and fight irrelevant people for irrational ends, may not societies also?

Of these other procedures for solving ambivalence *displacement* is unquestionably the simplest. It solves the emotional conflict which arises when you feel hatred for your friend by the simple expedient of deflecting the hatred and aggressive action to someone else, preferably someone smaller than yourself. Children constantly resort to it.

'Speaking to Dan, Mrs. I. called him " darling." Benjie at once said : " Why don't you call *me* that? " Mrs. I. replied : " But I often do." Benjie then said to Cecil : " I don't like you, Cecil. I'll get a gun and shoot you dead." '[1]

These children were both four years old, but Cecil was two months younger. Obviously to threaten Cecil had various advantages. Retaliation would be easier to deal with, remorse

[1] Isaacs, op. cit., p. 48.

would be absent and the friendly relation with Mrs. Isaacs uninterrupted.

A worried mother writes :

' My little girl, aged one year ten months, has become very difficult to manage owing, I expect, to jealousy, as she has a little brother of five months. At first she would hit him and start whining whenever I picked him up. I have not taken any notice of these fits, and never asked her to do anything for him, as I realized it only made her more angry. I am pleased to say this has been very effective, as she now asks to tuck him in, and mind him for me. She also offers him her toys, although she does not like parting with them. The real trouble now is that she absolutely refuses to have anything to do with strangers. If anyone says : " Good morning " or speaks to her at all, her reply is nearly always a very definite " No, don't " or " No, won't." She screams if they touch her or try to pick her up.'[1]

In this case it seems that the child has established an affectionate relation to the new baby by means of turning all her dislike on to other ' strangers.'

In older children dislike and criticism engendered by parental frustration is frequently vented upon school teachers. For instance, a child of eleven suffered from insomnia, listlessness and poor school work. On investigation it was found that the mother had always rejected this child and openly preferred her sister who was two years younger. The elder child, however, did not show open hostility to her mother. But after treatment had begun she began to criticize and laugh at her schoolmistress in a way which plainly showed it was an alternative to being antagonistic to her mother.

Displacements of this kind are equally common in adult life. Two instances have already been given of men who attacked the heads of their respective States. In neither case was there reason to suppose that the attackers had any rational grounds for their acts. In both cases there is an overwhelming probability that these men had displaced their hatred from someone nearer them, their father or their employer, for instance, on to the King or President. Actually this phenomenon is so common that it is taken for granted in everyday life. No one is surprised if a man who has been sacked from his job is in a bad temper and rude to his friends, or a girl who has been jilted takes an opportunity to lead on another man and then

---

[1] Isaacs, op. cit., p. 60.

jilt him. In the political sphere it is also commonly assumed. The idea that dictators undertake foreign adventures in order to deflect the people's resentment from themselves is not a psycho-analytic theory but an assumption of the common man. All that psycho-analysts have done has been to take these ideas seriously and try to understand them more thoroughly.

A good example of the displacement of aggression from its original target on to another was presented in a recent film (*Farewell Again*). It is a simple tale contrived to appeal to the ordinary man. Its assumption of the mechanism of displacement and its assumption that the ordinary cinema-goer will understand and accept it as a normal part of life seem to us eloquent testimony of the pervasiveness of displacement in social affairs.

A regiment is returning home after some years' service overseas. All the men are in high spirits in anticipation of seeing their wives, sweethearts or children again. Then as a bolt from the blue comes a message ordering them back to Palestine where disturbances are supposed to have broken out. The colonel does not seek to minimize the disappointment, but appeals to the men's sense of duty to carry out the order loyally. Most of them try to grin and bear it, but there is a feeling of injustice and much half-suppressed resentment at this sudden frustration of cherished dreams. The discontent grows, but except for one or two professional grumblers it is not directed against the colonel for whom the men have great affection, or even against the War Office. It remains rather aimless dissatisfaction manifesting itself in a variety of trifling ways. The men get on each other's nerves, old-standing feuds break out again, friends become irritable with one another. Finally two of the privates come to blows and a free fight follows throughout the mess. The colonel recognizing the source of the trouble makes another appeal for loyalty and makes every effort possible to ensure that the men will have as good a time as possible during the few hours in which the ship will be docked in England. Peace and discipline are restored.

In this story the men's anger resulting from the authorities' orders is not expressed directly. Partly perhaps from fear of punishment and partly because their sense of duty and loyalty to their colonel forbid it, these men are portrayed as suppressing their anger and avoiding mutiny. Yet their resentment persists and instead of being expressed against the people who were the cause of the frustration it is expressed against men who have had nothing whatever to do with it. The fight, instead of being between the men and the authorities, is between the men themselves. Their resentment has been displaced.

Although in most people the mechanisms of repression and displacement work tolerably well, fresh difficulties are apt to arise through the mechanism of control becoming hypertrophied. Just as we do not always confine ourselves to passive defence against an external murderer, so a person's conscience does not confine itself to reasonable control of his own murderous impulses. On the principle that attack is the best means of defence, a ruthless campaign is waged against condemned impulses with the object of extirpating them root and branch. When the controlling conscience develops such violent propensities towards the condemned impulses the internal conflict may become so unbearable that it demands relief. But before considering the methods whereby relief is obtained, methods which tend to produce much aggressive behaviour, it may be as well to explain how it is that a child's conscience becomes so violent.

Examples have already been given of the violent way in which children feel and behave towards a rival. The universal severity of their scales of punishment is its moral counterpart.

Their own parents and nurses may have been very tolerant towards their tempers and their greed and other childish vices. Yet they themselves are not satisfied with anything short of the utter extermination of evil. No schoolboy is content until the villain in a story has been hanged or shot, and girls are little more merciful. In schools where the children mete out punishments it is the usual experience of masters that the principal difficulty is in persuading the courts to be lenient.

No doubt children who have been severely treated for naughtiness will be more severe than others who have been tolerantly treated, but it is certain that children spontaneously conceive of punishments far more severe than those which they have either experienced or been threatened with. For instance, Isaacs quotes the case of ' a girl of three and a half years who asked her mother what would happen if she were naughty at school. Her mother said : " Well, what would ? " The child, after a pause, said : " I know—God would drown the world." '

Such phantasies are particularly common in neurotic children. While a rather nervous small girl of eight was playing, a cheap china doll fell off the table and was broken. The next time she came she was very afraid and it was not for a long time that she could be induced to leave her mother and play at all. When finally she did so, she pretended that there was a little girl who had broken her doll and had to be shot. Whereupon the tin soldiers were made to aim at her. When asked if she could be let off, she refused absolutely, saying that the little girl had been naughty in breaking her doll and must be punished. Her mother subsequently said that the child had been very upset on returning home the previous time, had constantly worried about the broken doll and had been extremely reluctant to come again.

The presence of such violent conceptions of punishment in children's minds comes as a shock. Yet it is only to be expected. Children are naturally violent. They do not do things by halves. When they love they do so with great generosity, when they hate they are not satisfied until their enemy is dead. And so with their scale of punishments. Because a child thinks that another should be whipped for being dirty or shot for breaking her doll, we need not assume that he or she has been cruelly treated at home. It is simply the expression of childish violence in the moral sphere.

These examples show moreover that children are ruthless towards evil in themselves as well as in others. The child whose doll was broken was not only afraid of being shot, but clearly felt she deserved it. Self-dissatisfaction over the performance of some mechanical task has already been emphasized (p. 68) as the cause of much ill-temper. Self-dissatisfaction in the moral sphere is no less important a cause. In each case feelings of anger are aroused, which may take the form of self-hatred or deliberate self-punishment with the object of purging the self of all ' bad ' impulses. The practice of self-flagellation to overcome and root out evil is out of fashion at present, widely though it was practised in the past. None the less much illness and many accidents prove on investigation to be due to a strong, usually unconscious, urge to punish the self, and suicide usually has this as one of its motives.[1]

Self-love and self-pity are such common conceptions that it is interesting that self-hatred should be so little recognized.

[1] Frequently the bad impulses which self-flagellation is intended to exterminate are dramatized and thought of by the sufferer as due to his having within him a devil or wild animal. The self-punishment is then directed against the ' introjected objects ' as these products of phantasy are termed. The super-ego may also be personalized, often in the character of a parent. This ' introjected parent ' may then be attacked instead of the real external person.

Further discussion of the problems arising from introjection has been omitted because of the desire to present psycho-analytic theory in its simplest possible form.

It is extraordinary how early tendencies to vent dissatisfaction upon the self manifest themselves ; the following letter from a mother testifies to its existence in the second year.

' My little boy is one year nine months old. He is very healthy and full of life, but if crossed in any way, such as not allowed to go out when any one comes to the door, if his engine turns over, or if checked for doing wrong, he gets down on his knees and bangs his forehead on the floor several times as hard as possible, or against the wall. He must hurt himself as he cries.'[1]

Now it is obvious from these examples that it is a very terrible thing for children to feel dissatisfied with themselves or guilty over anything. The tortures of a medieval Hell are no longer believed in by rational people, but observation shows that such ideas spring afresh in the irrational mind of every child. It is not only the vengeance of an angry and cruel God which is feared ; the more immediate punishments of an angry and cruel conscience are equally frightening. As a result of this overwhelming fear of punishment a strong motive arises for turning a blind eye to our own incapacities and moral shortcomings and seeing all that is weak, foolish and evil in others. In our own eyes we then cease to be the enemies of ourselves and of those we love, and see ourselves as the noble champions of all that is good against the follies and malevolence that other men contemplate.

This process of solving the conflict between condemning conscience and condemned impulses by seeing the mote in the other man's eye is known as *projection*.[1] The condemned impulses are projected and viewed as though they originated in someone else's heart. Internal conflict is thereby resolved and instead of self-reproach and suicidal feelings, there are feelings of saving the world from some vicious foe. The conflict goes on, but the enemy is someone else and can be vanquished without exterminating the self.

Innumerable instances could be given both from childhood and adult life.

Sometimes projection is confined to merely blaming another person. For instance :

In close succession a woman loses her mother and younger

---

[1] Isaacs, op. cit., p. 186.

[2] It is generally believed that the origin of projection lies in an infant including in its feeling of ' self ' all pleasant things which do its will, and excluding from its feeling of ' self ' all painful things which fail to do what it wants. In the interests of simplicity this theory and also the relation of projection to excretory functions have not been discussed in detail.

brother, both of whom she has had to nurse through long and painful illnesses. She has worked night and day for them, but has always felt her ministrations were insufficient. At the funerals relations talk and laugh, and the full blast of the girl's self-condemnations alight on their heads. *They* are unfeeling, *they* did nothing to help her during the illness, *they* regard the funeral as a joke. They are blameworthy, not she.

At other times more active measures are taken against the alleged malefactors.

The baby of a charwoman gets diphtheria. Someone must be blamed. Her landlord is slovenly and has many times refused to improve the house. He is, therefore, made the scapegoat ; the diphtheria is blamed on to the bugs in the house, and the mother gets the sanitary inspector on to the landlord.

A man has a motor accident in which he knocks down an old woman. He immediately begins to feel dissatisfied with the car and exchanges it within the week for a new one. Responsibility for the accident has been placed on the car.

Actual violence is by no means infrequent.

For instance a boy of nine had become very troublesome at school on account of his aggressive behaviour, hitting the other children about for no apparent reason and swearing. Whilst playing with some tin soldiers, he began shooting them with a pop-gun. On being asked who one soldier was, he said : " That's Colin Carver. He's a bad boy." Asked why, he said : " He hits the other boys and uses dirty words."

Another boy of seven also began shooting lead soldiers. On asking whom they represented, he replied : " That's Leslie Mathews. He's a dirty boy. He swears and pinches the other kiddies' things—and he's always smoking." This boy had been a persistent pilferer for several years and had recently taken to using bad language and smoking. Other children would not make friends with him because of his tendency to hit them.

Both of these incidents occurred at their first visit to a psychiatrist, and no suggestions of any kind had been made to them.

In each case we are probably quite safe in concluding that their aggressive behaviour at school was similar to their aggressive behaviour in play. They make the other children into scapegoats and then attack them.

Now this is a very important conclusion. Much aggressive behaviour in children, especially bullying, appears at first sight to be senseless. Yet careful investigation goes to show that these apparently senseless assaults have a perfectly logical origin. The child or person feels terribly guilty about something he has done or wished to do, then finds someone else to blame it on and finally attacks them for it. It is a procedure quite analogous to the bad temper which people get into with others when they themselves have done something stupid. An example has already been given of a boy who, having forgotten his ticket, flew into a rage with his mother and hit his brother. Many others could be given of golfers who, having missed an easy shot, get angry and vent it upon their wives on returning home ' because tea is late '.

The *need* for a scapegoat[1] is always to alleviate intolerable feelings of self-dissatisfaction and guilt. It may be remarked, however, that the *choice* is often the result of more realistic factors. The charwoman blames her bad landlord. The man blames the car which actually did the damage. The ' bad ' boys blame others who were no doubt also guilty. Such objects of course are always to hand for there are blemishes in everyone. The result is righteous indignation. We can go into tantrums of rage with people whose sins are small and thereby conveniently overlook shortcomings in ourselves which we fear are enormous. Campaigns of righteous indignation are often carried to preposterous lengths. Indeed, it is probably true that of all anger, righteous anger is the most ruthless, the most cruel and consequently the most dangerous. The result is always an utterly irrational attack upon someone who has in no wise deserved it. But, as has just been emphasised, the irrationality does nothing to mitigate the violence of the assault. It is because of this that psychoanalysts, when considering the most ruthless forms of group fighting—war—have kept their eyes open for manifestations of projection and scapegoat-hunting. As Glover[2] has pointed out, it is extremely probable that motives of this kind play a large part in war. In later sections we shall see that there is plenty of evidence to support such anticipations.

The projection of condemned impulses and feelings upon others is only one of the methods whereby the internal conflict between the condemning conscience and ' bad ' impulses can be solved. In this case the conscious self identifies itself with the conscience and sees the ' bad ' impulses in others. The alternative is for the conscious self to identify with the

---

[1] We are using the term ' scapegoat ' in this wide sense since it is used so colloquially. Strictly speaking perhaps it should be confined to procedures, such as the Jewish ritual in which personal sin is admitted and then placed upon some other creature to be borne away.

[2] Glover, *War, Sadism, and Pacifism*. Allen & Unwin, 1933.

condemned impulses and to see the condemnation coming from without. This process is known technically as the *projection of the super-ego.* Like the projection of ' bad ' impulses it leads to much aggression.

For instance, it was probably a motive in the incident already quoted in which Benjie, having accidentally broken a jug, became defiant and shouted : " I'll hit you in the face ; I'll not come to school any more." No punishment had been threatened and experience might have shown him that none was likely, yet like the little girl who was afraid that God would drown the world if she was naughty, Benjie anticipated some serious revenge. As a result, to protect himself from a danger which was almost entirely the product of his imagination. he became aggressive and threatened to attack.

The boy quoted on pp. 69–70 also showed this reaction. One day, whilst helping to clear the table, he smashed a coffee-pot. He thereupon threw some other crockery on the floor, got into a violent temper with his mother, who up till then had no idea what had happened, and began threatening her with a knife. From the boy's point of view this attack was simply self-defence. Unlike Benjie, he had been beaten a good deal so that his fears of punishment were not wholly imaginary. Nevertheless, analysis revealed that his conceptions of punishment were of an altogether fantastic severity, and he had come to expect them from people who in fact wished him nothing but well.

The motive of self-defence in aggressive behaviour requires especial emphasis. Mrs. Isaacs has observed that ' most of the aggressive behaviour of small children has a considerable element of defence about it,' and psycho-analysis has been able to explain it. The projection either of ' bad ' impulses or of the punishing super-ego leads in different ways to irrational fears of being attacked and consequently to unnecessary attacks in self-defence.

The tendency to project all one's own ' bad ' impulses on to others has the effect of turning friendly people into enemies in the imagination of the projector. A person with strong murderous impulses is apt, through projection, to see every one else as a potential murderer. A person who is inclined to bully will, through projection, see every one else as a bully. It is not he who wants to murder or to bully others ; they want to murder or bully him.

The projection of a condemning conscience equally leads to the belief that others are our enemies when in fact they may be friendly. Examples have just been given of children who, fearing severe punishment, attacked in self-defence. Examples could also be given of adults who, without realizing it, still anticipate punishment and revenge of the same devastating kind as they did when they were children. This may be disputed, yet we need only recall that at one time all intelligent people and even now very large numbers consciously believe that the vilest tortures await them in Hell in punishment for wrong-doing. Again, patients in a melancholia are always afraid of the most terrible punishments such as being thrown to lions or being cut to pieces, fears which can be nothing but products of their own guilty imaginations. With these facts in mind it is less difficult to believe that fears of a fantastic kind may also be present in the minds of ordinary people, despite their consciously disowning them, and account for the remarkable guiltiness with which many people sense criticism and, in self-defence, attack the critic.

In these ways imaginary enemies of an extraordinary malevolence are created. (It is now believed that all the phobias and other terrors of neurotics are to be explained in this way.) The effect of such fears upon social life is, of course, tremendous and almost entirely for ill. The natural rivalry and distrust of children is quite sufficient without any added complications. There is ample real enmity without imaginary enmity. It is hardly surprising, therefore, that with the added strain upon friendship imposed by projection, peaceful co-operation quickly breaks down ; nor that many fights are undertaken in the genuine though mistaken belief that other people are attacking.

Conclusions.

We may now summarize the contribution which psycho-analysis has made to the understanding of hatred and aggression :

(1) It has drawn attention to the existence of *unconscious aggressive impulses* which influence people's behaviour without their being aware of the fact.

(2) It has emphasized the role which *ambivalence*, the tendency to love and hate the same person, plays in personal relations, and explored the situations which give rise to this paradoxical state of affairs. Frustrations at the breast, jealousy over the birth of a new baby, and also of the affectionate relations between the two parents are amongst its most important sources.

(3) The universal *violence* of children's feelings is stressed, especially as this violence tends to persist unconsciously in adult life.

(4) The desire to consolidate friendships and to abhor ambivalent relations has been found to give rise to various dodges for disguising and disowning unfriendly impulses such as hatred and greed.

(5) Of these, *repression* was the first to be discovered. Unwanted impulses are banished from consciousness although this does not always result in their immobilization.

(6) Another procedure designed to solve the conflict of ambivalence is *displacement*. Here the impulse is permitted expression, but the object is changed. Instead of feeling angry and hurting a friend, we feel angry with and hurt a stranger. The result is an entirely irrational act of aggression.

(7) Feelings of shame and guilt over certain impulses lead to intense self-condemnation and self-hatred and the fear of terrible punishments. Such feelings are often unbearable and demand alleviation. This is found in two ways :

(*a*) *The condemned impulses are projected,* namely, attributed to someone else. These others, the scapegoats, are then seen as wicked people full of murderous and other evil wishes which must be stamped out.

(*b*) Alternatively *the condemning super-ego is projected.* Again the person will feel guiltless, but will view the people upon whom he has projected his super-ego as cruel oppressors.

(8) Projection, either of 'bad' impulses or of the conscience, has the effect of creating imaginary enemies, people of untold wickedness and malevolence, who are felt to be threatening our friends or ourselves. Much aggression is undertaken in self-defence against these imaginary enemies.

(4) ANIMISM

We have now completed our survey of the situations in which outbursts of aggression occur in the individual. But before discussing the theory of group-aggression to which these and other observations lead us, a further deep-rooted tendency of the human mind to which both anthropology and psycho-analysis have drawn attention needs description. This is the widespread tendency of people to attribute a personal motivation to every event which affects them, whatever its actual origin. Primitive peoples have long been known to hold such views. Frazer's *Golden Bough* is full of examples of the way in which savages attribute misadventures and calamities of all kinds to the deliberate malevolence of some being or other.

And not only does the savage blame the spirits for all the trouble that befalls him ; he attacks them.

' Their constant presence wearies him, their sleepless malignity exasperates him ; he longs with an unspeakable longing to be rid of them altogether, and from time to time, driven to bay, his patience utterly exhausted, he turns fiercely on his persecutors and makes a desperate effort to chase the whole pack of them from the land, to clear the air of their swarming multitudes, that he may breathe more freely and go on his way unmolested, at least for a time. Thus it comes about that the endeavour of· primitive people to make a clean sweep of all their troubles generally takes the form of a grand hunting out and expulsion of devils or ghosts. They think that if they can only shake off these their accursed tormentors, they will make a fresh start in life, happy and innocent ; the tales of Eden and the old poetic golden age will come true again.'[1]

Innumerable examples of the manner in which primitives seek to exterminate their supposed persecutors, the demons and spirits who cause sickness, drought, typhoon and all the other disasters man is heir to, are given in the *Golden Bough*.

' Some of the native tribes of Central Queensland believe in a noxious being called Molonga, who prowls unseen and would kill men and violate women if certain ceremonies were not performed. These ceremonies last for five nights and consist of dances, in which only men, fantastically painted and adorned, take part. On the fifth night Molonga himself, personified by a man tricked out with red ochre and feathers and carrying a long feather-tipped spear, rushes forth from the darkness at the spectators and makes as if he would run them through. Great is the excitement, loud are the shrieks and shouts, but after another feigned attack the demon vanishes in the gloom.'[2]

' In the Island of Rook, between New Guinea and New Britain, when any misfortune has happened, all the people run together, scream, curse, howl, and beat the air with sticks to drive away the devil, who is supposed to be the author of the mishap. From the spot where the mishap took place they drive him step by step to the sea, and on reaching the shore they redouble their shouts and blows in order to expel him from the island. He generally retires to the sea or to the Island of Lottin.'[3]

[1] *The Golden Bough*, abridged edition, p. 547.
[2] Op. cit., pp. 562–3.
[3] Op. cit., p. 547.

' When a village has been visited by a series of disasters or a severe epidemic, the inhabitants of Minahassa in Celebes lay the blame upon the devils who are infesting the village and who must be expelled from it. Accordingly, early one morning all the people, men, women, and children, quit their homes, carrying their household goods with them, and take up their quarters in temporary huts which have been erected outside the village. Here they spend several days, offering sacrifices and preparing for the final ceremony. At last the men, some wearing masks, others with their faces blackened, and so on, but all armed with swords, guns, pikes, or brooms, steal cautiously and silently back to the deserted village. Then, at a signal from the priest, they rush furiously up and down the streets and into and under the houses (which are raised on piles above the ground), yelling and striking on walls, doors, and windows, to drive away the devils. Next the priests and the rest of the people come with the holy fire and march nine times round each house and thrice round the ladder that leads up to it, carrying the fire with them. Then they take the fire into the kitchen, where it must burn away, and great and general is the joy.'[1]

This conviction of universal human motivation is usually known as *animism*.[2] It is far less explicit in the civilized person than it is in the savage and therefore less easy to demonstrate. The absurdity of the savage's views on the causes of storms or disease is obvious to westerners, but, since no one likes to admit the absurdities of his own beliefs, it is difficult to convince a European that his also are often animistic. Nevertheless we believe animism to be fully as important in civilized societies as in primitive. It is not so long since everyone in Western Europe believed that all events emanated either from God or the Devil. It is true that such explanations are out of fashion now, but even to-day many religious people still believe that health and prosperity, sickness and disaster are equally dependent on God's will. The law itself enshrines the belief in the words ' Act of God '. But now that science and rationalism have largely discredited the belief in super-human agencies it might be expected that animism would die altogether. This does not appear to be the case. What

---

[1] Fraser, op. cit., p. 548.

[2] The term 'animism' is sometimes confined to the attribution of souls or minds to inanimate objects. We think it legitimate, however, to extend the term to cover all instances where phenomena believed nowadays to be of non-human origin are attributed to the workings of human or para-human wills. The agents which can be held responsible fall into three classes : (1) spirits, demons, etc. ; (2) other human beings ; (3) the person's own self.

happens is that the tendency to attribute blame to someone continues, but that instead of its being attached to spirits it becomes attached to other groups of men. For instance, in September 1867 ' the inhabitants of Calabria (Spain), imagining the cholera to be occasioned by poison, murder whole families on suspicion of scattering it ; eighty persons are cut to pieces and thrown to the swine.'[1] A similar belief, that death is always due to murder, was expressed by a small boy of five. He made a comment about the King being shot and on being questioned remarked : " Well, we've got a new King now. I suppose a soldier must have shot the other one." Many further examples of this, both from primitive and civilized societies, are given in the sections on group aggression.

It seems probable that the tendency to see a human agency at work behind all natural phenomena is initially a simple intellectual error—a false explanation deriving from inadequate knowledge. Psycho-analysis has demonstrated, however, that the intellectual error is reinforced by the strong emotional forces which have already been discussed. The human agencies deemed responsible are not conceived of as either capricious or uninterested. On the contrary their every act is believed to be inspired by personal motives such as love or revenge, a desire to reward or a lust to punish. Thus plentiful crops and fertile women are not simply good fortune. They are the intentional reward for good behaviour. Storms, tempest and earthquake are likewise either malicious revenge or deliberate punishment for evil. This idea is so well known as hardly to need illustration, but it is interesting to hear it expressed apparently spontaneously by a boy of four.

' The children were standing at the door, watching a heavy shower of rain. They heard the rustling noise of the rain on the leaves, and when something was said about this, George remarked : " Perhaps it's God saying He will punish us for doing things we shouldn't." ' [2]

So far we have only mentioned cases in which the misfortune is attributed to some external being, a spirit or God or the malice of other men. Almost all the anthropological observations are of this kind. Psycho-analytic research has emphasized another aspect. It is frequently found that people hold *themselves* responsible for calamities with which they have in fact had nothing to do. We all know people who like to

---

[1] Quoted from *Marshall's Ladies' Fashionable Repository* for 1869 in *The Times*, 12 June 1937.
[2] Isaacs, op. cit., p. 172.

take the *credit* for everything that happens, whether they are really responsible or not. Such a motive is easily understood. What is not so often recognized is that people are just as apt to take the *blame* for events which they have not really influenced at all. Naturally they do not shout about it so much, indeed they are inclined to deny it to themselves as well as to others, but an enormous amount of evidence has now accumulated to show that people frequently feel responsible for natural misfortunes, often without realizing that they are holding themselves so.[1]

The illness or death of a relative is one of the most frequent sources of such guilt, as the following case-histories illustrate.

A small boy of seven was brought for advice by his mother, because of disobedience, tempers, teasing and hurting two little sisters. On investigation it was found that he had been fairly easy to manage until a sister was born, when he was three years old. He had shown intense jealousy of the new arrival and from that time onwards outbursts of rage would follow any frustration, particularly over food.[2] He would go tense, sometimes threatened to kill the baby, sometimes punched his mother. After these outbursts he became very affectionate and showed great concern for them both. (Similar cases to this abound. A simple situation of frustration and jealousy gives rise to acute anger and aggression towards both the rival new-comer and the traitor mother. This is badly handled and, instead of settling down, becomes a chronic condition. Outbursts of rage and aggression follow any new situation of rivalry and frustration.) But the boy is still genuinely fond of his mother and the outbursts of anger are followed by remorse, thus illustrating that such feelings are born, not of a conventional morality imposed from without, but of simple feelings of affection and a natural desire to be nice to those most loved. Later on his mother fell ill. His remorse then became specially pronounced. He promised again and again that he would never more be naughty and hurt her and, when she was in hospital, made daily pilgrimages to see how she was. On the days when visitors were not allowed

---

[1] Usually when no conscious feelings of guilt are experienced, the person suffers from a sense of inferiority, a feeling of not being liked, or from depression when misfortunes occur. Psycho-analysts are sometimes ridiculed for talking about an ' unconscious sense of guilt,' but it should be remembered that it is an old religious conception. Although not actually experiencing guilt, these people are very touchy if criticized and often become aggressive.

[2] Food is of double importance to children. Not only are they greedy and like it, but food is part of their earliest relation with their mother. A simple jealousy situation of great intensity results from seeing another child being suckled.

in he would walk around the hospital in the hope of catching a glimpse of her at the window. Naturally he was enormously relieved when she recovered.

This boy's behaviour during his mother's illness, especially his promising gratuitously never to hurt her again, showed plainly that he was blaming himself for her condition. Such self-reproach is in fact unjustified, because, of course, the boy was in no way the cause of his mother's illness. But children have not adult knowledge of cause and effect. All this boy knew was that there had been times when he had punched his mother and wanted to kill her. When she fell ill a guilty conscience led him to conclude that he was the cause of it.

This description was given to me by the mother and was not the result of psycho-analysis, but similar processes are revealed with extraordinary regularity during the analyses of even quite normal adults and children. *Events which happen to be in accordance with aggressive wishes are assumed to have been caused by those wishes.* This erroneous but extremely common conclusion is the result partly of the widespread tendency towards animism which holds that all events are of human or para-human origin, and partly to another fundamental tendency of the human mind, the tendency to equate wish and deed. This latter tendency, known technically as the *omnipotence of thought*, is found in all children and is a characteristic of the obsessional neurotic. These patients are terrified that if they think a thing it will happen, and since their thoughts are usually of a horrifying character, either murderous or obscene, they undergo great torment fighting them. Naturally they are particularly prone to shoulder responsibilities which do not really belong to them. It is from their ranks that the miserable individuals are recruited who, when a murder has been committed, straightway go to the police and confess to having done it.

Dr. Karin Stephen[1] has described a case in which the assumption that an event which is in accordance with aggressive wishes has actually been caused by those wishes is particularly clear, and was at the root of a serious mental breakdown.

Miss M. had suffered all her life from the idea that she was like Cain, the murderer of Abel. She had also a great horror of jealousy and did her utmost to avoid ever feeling jealous of any one. She was unmarried and lived with her mother, being the typical self-sacrificing daughter, continually making her mother presents and taking great care of her health. She spoke in a timid innocent voice, was entirely submissive to

---

[1] Stephen, *Psycho-Analysis and Medicine.*

everyone and undertook all the housework whilst her younger sister studied and earned prizes. At the age of thirty she had a breakdown, during which she turned against her mother and accused her of having ruined her life.

This was her history as she remembered it during psychoanalysis :

'When she was nearly four her mother had another baby and she, as the elder child, was turned out of her cot in the parents' bedroom by its arrival. The day after the new baby was born she was allowed to go in and see her mother, and asked if she might hold the baby, but in a few moments she begged the nurse to take it from her because she felt sure she was going to drop it. Next day the baby died. This did not seem to her a mere coincidence : she appears to have believed that she was in some way responsible. It was undoubtedly true that she had wished the new baby might be removed, and now, when it did, in fact, die, she felt as if the wish had *brought this about*. She got back her cot in her parents' bedroom and remembers feeling glad but guilty at being there again. She said she tried to believe what they told her, that it was the fault of the nurse who had let the baby get a chill, but she knew she had been frightfully jealous, and the idea haunted her that somehow her jealousy had killed it. . . .

'Four years after the death of this baby her mother had another, which once again turned the elder child out of her cot in her parents' room. She remembers being in the top room with her doll, and first trying to kiss it and be fond of it, then getting angry with it and pushing its eyes in. She was frightened when she had done that, and tried to get the eyes back again, but she could not. Finally she slid the doll to the edge of the bed and succeeded in having it fall out on the floor without *exactly* having pushed it. . . .

'Later, when she had to wheel out the new baby in the pram, she contrived, in spite of strict warnings to avoid pavements, that the wheels mounted on the curb crookedly, the pram overturned, and the baby fell into the road. This time, fortunately, the baby did not die.

'She had never connected her terrible feelings of being like Cain and her over-powering dread of jealousy with these episodes.'

This latter case is specially interesting as demonstrating how hatred can develop from feelings of overwhelming guilt over an incident in which the person had not actually had any hand. The train of events may be schematized thus :

(1) The new baby dies.

(2) Someone must be responsible (animism).

(3) Because she has wished the baby to die the child holds herself responsible (omnipotence of thought).

(4) To assuage the guilt and make amends to the mother the child's conscience demands great self-sacrifice.

(5) Self-sacrifice is so great that life becomes intolerable.

(6) Instead of rebelling against her own severe conscience the girl projects all responsibility for her miserable life on to her mother (projection of super-ego) and accuses her of ruining her life.

It is found in clinical practice that accusations of this kind are often the prelude to physical assaults.

Similar feelings of guilt over a death quite unconnected with the patient were observed after the death of King George. One girl of twenty, with pronounced hatred towards both her parents, was very depressed the following day and said she had had a recurrent self-accusatory thought the previous evening when the King was dying : 'You killed the King.' Dr. Fairbairn reported the case of a youth of eighteen whose symptoms of anxiety turned into panic at each wireless bulletin. During the night following that on which the King died, he dreamt that he had shot a man representing his father. Later in the dream he heard shouts which seemed to come from the person whom he had killed ; but this person now seemed to be his brother (who was six years younger than the patient and died aged six). Similar evidence made it quite clear that he had always felt responsible for his younger brother's death and that these feelings of guilt had been reactivated by the King's death.

Ordinary clinical and also psycho-analytic observations thus explain how it is that people can come to feel guilty over and blame themselves for occurrences with which, in fact, they have had nothing whatever to do. There are few people who do not have some such feelings of guilt connected with their fantasies of destruction. They may remain dormant for long periods but are aroused afresh by actual disasters, such as the death of a relative or a national misfortune.

Now it is when people feel most guilty themselves that they are most apt either to find fault with others (projection of ' bad ' impulses), or to interpret every event that is disadvantageous to themselves as being deliberate punishment (projection of super-ego), against which they must protect

themselves. Consequently large numbers of people after they
or their friends have suffered adversity become truculent and
bellicose. This sequence is well illustrated by the following
incident.

> 'Dan (4.8) and Priscilla (6.5) said they would "push
> Phineas (2.11) to make him cry again." When they were
> going to him again, Mrs. I. held them back and would not
> let them go near him, and in trying to run past Mrs. I.,
> Christopher (5.4) bumped his head on the door. The
> others thought Mrs. I. had done this to him, and were very
> angry, saying that she was "horrid and beastly," and "we
> shan't come to tea with you any more." Priscilla said :
> "Let's be rude to her," and made threatening faces at her.
> When presently they understood that she had not done it to
> Christopher, they calmed down and were friendly.'

Here Dan and Priscilla had been actively hostile to a younger
child. Mrs. Isaacs interfered and the two children evidently
felt guilty. Then an irrelevant accident happens to another
child. In their guilty frame of mind Dan and Priscilla fear
they are responsible ; it is consequently a great relief to them
to fix the blame for it upon someone else. In the first place
they see hostility in someone else instead of in themselves
(projection of 'bad' impulses) ; in the second place, by fixing
it upon Mrs. Isaacs, they can discredit the very person who
made them feel guilty.

The tendency to incriminate an external being for natural
events is, therefore, seen to be as much due to a need to deny
personal guilt, and to find an external scapegoat, as to any
intellectual mistake. Were it not for the need to prove their
own innocence, they would not be so concerned to prove
someone else's guilt. This view is based largely on psycho-
analytic evidence, but anthropological observations confirm it.

In Frazer's descriptions of the tribes already quoted, there
is no hint that the tribesmen feel any guilt for the disaster,
blame for which they pin on the spirits. But there are others
who, before expelling the evil agents, confess their sins. The
Iroquois, for instance, actually had a general confession of
sins as part of the expulsion ceremony, which served, Frazer
says, as 'a way of stripping the people of their moral burdens,
that these might be collected and cast out.' The scapegoat
ceremony of the Jews seems to be a more civilized form of the
same process. 'On the Day of Atonement, which was the
tenth day of the seventh month, the Jewish high-priest laid

---

[1] Isaacs, op. cit., pp. 262–263.

both his hands on the head of a live goat, confessed over it all the iniquities of the Children of Israel, and, having thereby transferred the sins of the people to the beast, sent it away into the wilderness.'[1]

Frazer has no hesitation in grouping instances such as this where the community sense of guilt is admitted with those (quoted on pp. 95–6) where it appears absent. We are, therefore, probably safe in concluding that where the Jews admitted their own guilt and deliberately and consciously laid it upon another, the more primitive peoples, despite apparent guiltlessness, really do fear counting themselves responsible for disasters and are relieved by being able to blame the spirits.

In primitive warfare, the tendency to animism, coupled with a need to find someone else guilty, will be found to play a leading part. Indeed, no understanding of hostile behaviour in humans is possible, in our view, without constant reference to animism and projection. This is discussed at length on pages 117 to 123; meanwhile we may summarize our conclusions.

Conclusions.

(1) Events such as tempest or disease or economic depression, which are the common calamity of all, are always given a personal origin by children and primitive peoples. They thus become the sources of personal hatreds against spirits or humans.

(2) Animism, coupled with a primitive belief in the omnipotence of thought, tends to increase the sense of guilt, through people attributing to themselves calamities for which they are, in fact, in no way responsible. It has already been shown that an over-burdening sense of guilt is liable to lead, through projection, to accusations, and hostile behaviour. Animism, by increasing guilt, therefore stimulates hostile behaviour.

(3) Finally, animism plays into the hands of projection. Every calamity for which *we* are not responsible is an additional proof of the badness of *others*. When rain falls it confirms our belief in an angry punishing spirit or God. When crops fail it proves that the spirits or our neighbours are unpleasant and malevolent people. Animism, whilst on the one hand tending enormously to increase the sense of guilt, at the same time provides an excellent procedure for seeing the blame in others

---

[1] Frazer, op. cit., pp. 553 and 569.

and proving ourselves innocent. In so doing it vastly exaggerates the mutual fear and distrust in which people live.

B. STUDIES IN GROUP AGGRESSION

(1) WAR BETWEEN PRIMITIVE COMMUNITIES

It is the authors' contention that war is simply a particular example of fighting, and that in all probability the origins of fighting amongst groups will be substantially the same as the origins of fighting between individuals. It is now proposed to review the apparent causes of war amongst primitive communities to test out our hypothesis. In the space at our disposal it is impossible for this survey to be more than rough and general. Nor have we had an opportunity to examine the original anthropological descriptions. We are, in consequence, deeply indebted to Professor Davie for his invaluable collection and classification of it. What follows is largely based upon his work.[1]

All authorities who have studied the data seem to be agreed upon the extremely widespread incidence of warfare amongst the simpler peoples. Hobhouse, Wheeler, and Ginsberg examined the records of three hundred and eleven primitive societies, ranging from the lower hunters to those who have developed simple forms of agriculture. Amongst these they found an ' aggregate of two hundred and ninety-eight cases of war or feuds distributed through all the grades, and nine certain and four doubtful cases of " no war." These are mainly confined to the lowest grades, there being four and a half among the lower, three and a half among the higher hunters, and two in the lowest agriculture.'[2]

Davie writes : ' War plays a prominent part in the life of most primitive peoples and is usually a sanguinary affair,' and again, ' The cases where war is unknown or unimportant have been considered in some detail for the reason that they are quite exceptional.' And not only is it very exceptional to find societies where war is almost unknown, but of the warlike tribes there is actually a majority who live in a state of *continual* warfare. ' A survey of the primitive tribes existing to-day shows that those living in a continual state of war greatly outnumber those that are predominantly peaceful.' For example :

---

[1] Davie, *The Evolution of War*, Yale University Press, 1929.
[2] Hobhouse, Wheeler, and Ginsberg, *The Material Culture and Social Institutions of the Simpler Peoples*.

' Incessant warfare was the rule among the Eskimos and Indians of Alaska and the islands of the far north-west. The same was true of the Micmac Indians and the Beothucs of Newfoundland, between whom " there reigns so mortal an enmity that they never meet but a bloody conflict ensues." The tribes of Sitka Island are reported to be " perpetually in a state of warfare," while peace was the exception among the Salish tribes of British Columbia.

' The organization and distribution of the Indians of the United States resulted in a continual state of war. Each tribe was practically at war with every other tribe with which it did not have an express treaty of peace. A state of preparedness always existed, even when war was not actually in operation, and defensive works were often erected. War was intensified by the acquisition of firearms and the horse, and by the crowding back of tribe against tribe by the whites.' [1]

Nor is this warfare always of a mild nature.

' The evidence . . . .shows that thousands of persons have been slain in single battles among the African natives, that in America and elsewhere entire tribes have been exterminated, and that in certain South Sea Islands accumulated heaps of skull trophies cluster the beaches.'

Summing up Davie writes :

' Primitive tribes in general are more warlike than peaceful, and their warfare is severe and sanguinary more often than it is mild and bloodless. Nomadic races are as a rule more belligerent than agriculturists, and are more often engaged in war ; their constant wanderings in search of water and fresh grazing or hunting grounds lead to incessant conflicts with other tribes. As a corollary to this, mountain tribes are almost universally more warlike than those of the plains and valleys. The latter are generally agriculturists, since their land is more fertile, while the environment of the former is more suited to hunting and cattle raising. The conflict of herders and tillers, with the former dominating the latter, is a common phenomenon in culture history. Agricultural civilization, however, does not necessarily conduce to peace. On the contrary, with the growth of population and political control, war becomes more widespread and destructive. Thus the Aztecs of Mexico, the Incas of Peru, the African kingdoms of Dahomey and Benin,

---

[1] Davie, op. cit., p. 54.

and the ancient civilizations of Egypt, Babylonia, Assyria, and Persia all stand out as more militaristic than the less civilized tribes about them. Encounters were on a larger scale, and effective conquest now for the first time became feasible.'[1]

Despite this overwhelming evidence, the fact that there are some very simple peoples where war seems to be unknown has given rise to assertions that man is 'essentially' peaceful, and that it is civilization which is to blame for his present undeniable aggressiveness. Ginsberg has dealt at length with this theory.[2]

'Several anthropologists have recently advocated what amounts to a return to the myth of a golden age of innocence and peace on the ground that the simplestp eoples, namely the hunters and food-gatherers, are, it is alleged, gentle and peaceful. I refer to the school of Pater Schmidt in Germany, of Prof. Elliot Smith and Dr. Perry in England, and of Bij in Holland. As an argument in favour of pacifism this is a double-edged weapon ; for the believers in warfare may retort that these peoples remained in their primitive condition just because they could not or would not fight, and that war is essential to civilization. This has in fact been urged by Steinmetz. In any event the facts when closely scrutinized do not really justify any belief in the essential peacefulness of primitive man. The antithesis between war and peace is really inapplicable to the simple conditions in which these peoples live. Anything like the organized and aggressive warfare which we find in early history and among the more advanced of the simpler societies can have no place in the life of the simplest societies, for this implies organization, discipline, and differentiation between leaders and led which the people of the lowest culture do not possess. But if these do not have war, neither have they peace. We must think of war not as a genus uniquely opposed to peace, but as a species of violence opposed to social order and security. Scrutiny of the evidence shows that there are singularly few peoples among whom violence, homicidal and other, is unknown. This seems to be true of some of the Semang. The Veddas of recent times do not fight, but formerly they used to kill trespassers and eat their livers (for constancy in revenge). The Kubu do not fight, but the groups avoid each other and hardly ever meet. The Australian

---

[1] Davie, op. cit., p. 63.
[2] Ginsberg, *A Symposium on the Psychology of Peace and War.* *British Journal of Medical Psychology, XIV.*

tribes have no war in the sense of collective fighting by whole tribes, but there is or was a widespread system of vengeance against members of other groups and retaliation within the group. This is mitigated by the machinery of ordeals and the regulated combat, but this machinery is no doubt inspired and sustained by the serious possibility of feuds and homicide. Murder by magic and the fear of such murders constitute an important factor in Australian life. Fighting between groups on questions of trespass and personal injury is reported for the Andaman Islanders, the Ona, the Botocudo, the Bushmen. Among the Yaghans of Tierra del Fuego there were feuds between banded families, and concerted revenge occurs among the Punans and the Batua Pygmies. In such feuds the groups may not be involved as wholes, and perhaps the term war ought to be confined to such collective fighting. It would seem that war in this sense grows with the consolidation of groups and economic development. Among the simplest peoples we ought to speak rather of feuds, and these unquestionably occur on grounds of abduction of women, or resentments of trespass or personal injury. It must be conceded that these societies are peaceful by comparison with the more advanced of the primitive peoples. But violence and fear of violence are there and fighting occurs, though that is obviously and necessarily on a small scale.'

It seems then that the most primitive peoples are not only not peaceable, but live in a state not far removed from that of baboons. This has already been commented upon. The groups consist of only a few families and are bound together neither by rules nor institutions. Fights and feuds occur, but remain private ; the group as a whole does not combine together in an attack. As Ginsberg says, this state cannot be described as either peace or war, any more than a baboon community or a group of children can be said to be at peace or at war. For peace implies an absence of fighting and seems to require rules for its maintenance whilst war demands combined actions of one group against another.

Such primitive communities are rare. The great majority of primitive peoples live in larger groups and these are all characterized by the presence of rules regulating conduct. But whatever groups we study it seems to be taken for granted that members of it should treat fellow-members and strangers completely differently. In fact two codes of conduct appear, one prescribing a man's behaviour towards members of his own group, another towards strangers. The one is a code of peace, the other usually of war. Within the group, rights, laws, and institutions exist (such as bans on murder and stealing), obviously designed to settle disputes and promote peaceful relations between members. But not only do these rules exclude strangers, often customs exist which prescribe exactly opposite treatment for them.

'Against outsiders it is meritorious to kill, plunder, practise blood revenge, and steal women and slaves, but inside the group none of these things can be allowed. . . . The Sioux must kill a man before he can be a brave, and the Dyak before he can marry. Yet, as Tylor has said, " these Sioux among themselves hold manslaughter to be a crime unless in blood revenge ; and the Dyaks punish murder. . . . The tribe makes its law, not on an abstract principle that manslaughter is right or wrong, but for its own preservation. . . . Not only is slaying an enemy in open war looked on as righteous but ancient law goes on the doctrine that slaying one's own tribesman and slaying a foreigner are crimes of quite different order." '

' The Australian has two sets of mores, one for his group-comrades or friends, the other for outsiders or foes. "Between the males of a tribe there always exists a strong feeling of brotherhood, so that, come weal, come woe, a man can always calculate on the aid, in danger, of every member of his tribe," but toward strangers there reigns inveterate hatred, and any means are justified in dealing with them.'

' Captain Butler says that the Angami of North-East India are, among themselves, usually most truthful and honest ; against outsiders, however, they are " bloodthirsty, treacherous, and revengeful to an almost incredible degree." '[1]

In fact the higher savage civilizations are very similar to advanced Western civilizations in these respects. Within the group, members of each are comparatively peaceful and orderly. Towards other groups each shows undisguised suspicion and hostility. Practically the only difference between a European and a primitive in this respect is the variation in the size of the groups within which peace, law and co-operation reign and between which wars are waged.

The history of civilization can be viewed as a series of steps whereby organized social groups have expanded to

[1] Davie, op. cit., pp. 18–20.

contain more and more people. For civilized men living in nation states whose populations are measured in millions it is difficult to envisage the minute groups in which savages live. In New Guinea the native tribes are so segregated that ' twenty-five different languages are certainly spoken on the three hundred miles of coast extending from Yule Island to China Straits.'[1] This means that each group is on the average confined to twelve miles of coastline. A similar condition of affairs is found in the Naga Hills of India, in East Africa and many other places where the constant state of hostilities between neighbours has resulted in village communities becoming so socially isolated that they hardly understand one another's speech. Yet we have only to remember the small principalities and city-states of Europe or the persistent feuds between small Scottish clans up till comparatively recent times to realize how segregated social life has always tended to be.

This tendency of social groups to be peaceful within and war-like without is of critical interest. It will be remembered that observation on children reveal the large rôle which *displacement* plays in the development of their social life. In order to retain friends and consolidate peaceful relations, hatred for comrades, when aroused, has to be directed on to others. From what is known of the development of adult communities it is difficult not to conclude that displacement of aggression from friends to strangers has also played a major part in their development. The theory which we wish to put forward is that man, having so much of the baboon in his nature, has the greatest difficulty in living in peaceable and co-operative relations with his fellows in a group and that he is enabled to do so far more easily when he diverts his anti-social impulses against other groups. It is easier for him to avoid murdering his relatives and friends or stealing their wives if he has plenty of opportunity to murder other men and steal their wives.

If this theory is correct, internal peace and cohesion in a society is bought at the expense of waging wars on other groups just as the friendship of Benjie with Mrs. Isaacs necessitated hostilities against Cecil. In other words primitive man, by the process of displacement, exchanged a cat and dog existence in which there were numerous private feuds and every man's hand was against every other for a civilised existence in which peace within and war without reigned inseparable like Siamese Twins.

[1] Quoted by Davie, op. cit., p. 15.

Although the historical and comparative evidence all points to displacement having played a critical part in the establishment of social groups, peaceful within and war-like without, there is, so far as we know, no direct evidence to prove it. There can be no such doubt about the rôle of projection however. Just as in Europe, it is invariable for primitive groups to exalt themselves at the expense of foreigners. Anthropologists have termed it ' ethnocentrism.'

' " Each group," says Sumner, " nourishes its own pride and vanity, boasts itself superior, exalts its own divinities, and looks with contempt on outsiders. Each group thinks its own folkways the only right ones, and if it observes that other groups have other folkways, these excite its scorn. Opprobrious epithets are derived from these differences. ' Pig-eater,' ' cow-eater,' ' uncircumcised,' ' jabberers,' are epithets of contempt and abomination." ' [1]

Leonard Woolf reports : '_Over and over again have I been told by a villager in the jungle districts of Ceylon that the inhabitants of the neighbouring village, five or six miles away, were " bad people "—yet they were all of the same race, caste, and religion, had probably to some extent inter-married, and to the eye of an outsider were morally indistinguishable."[2]

This tendency to attribute all good qualities to one's own group and all bad qualities to others has even influenced the naming of different tribes. It has been shown that the names which primitive peoples give themselves when examined are mostly found to mean ' men,' implying that ' we alone are men ' and that the others are not real men. The name given to a neighbouring tribe may even imply rank abuse.

' The term Inuit, applied by the Eskimos to themselves, means " men " or " people ". The word Eskimo itself is derived from an Algonquian term meaning " eaters of raw flesh ". The Greenland Eskimos think that Europeans have been sent to Greenland to learn virtue and good manners from them. " Their highest form of praise for a European is that he is, or soon will be, as good as a Greenlander." '

' The Narimyeri of South Australia call themselves " men ", and designate all other tribes as " Merkam "—wild or savage. Where a distinction is drawn between tribesmen and aliens, the term applied to the latter is usually one of contempt or of fear. Thus the Kurnai speak of themselves as " men ", and give the name of Brajerak, from

[1] Quoted by Davie, op. cit., p. 22.   [2] Woolf, *Quack Quack*!

bra, " man," and *jerak,* " rage," or " anger," to certain
of their neighbours. They call the people who live in the
Western Port district of Victoria, Thurung or " tiger-
snakes ", because " they came sneaking about to kill us." ' [1]

The Jews of the Old Testament regarded themselves as the
Chosen People, their God as the only God, and all other
peoples, such as the Philistines and Amalekites, as so much
dross.

This attitude towards strangers is further exemplified by the
use of the same word for stranger and enemy. Tylor writes :
' The old state of things is well illustrated in the Latin word
hostis, which, meaning originally stranger, passed quite
naturally into the sense of enemy.' The conviction that
every stranger is an enemy reminds us also of children's
behaviour. It seems probable that in each case there is both
fear of possible rivalry coupled with the fear resulting from
projecting all that is evil on to him. Whatever the explanation
there is no doubt about the resulting behaviour.

' Curr writes of the native Australians : " Strangers
invariably look on each other as deadly enemies," and the
Australians never neglect " to massacre all strangers who
fall into their power." What Von Pfeil says of the Kanaka
of Bismarck Archipelago applies also to the Melanesians in
general. " Any person," he writes, " from a village removed
beyond the small district which the Kanaka looks upon as
his home he considers a stranger, and consequently an
enemy." Existence is so insecure outside of one's own group
that " no Kanaka may, without risk of life, attempt to visit
the district of a tribe with which his own is not on distinctly
friendly terms." '

' Even among the peaceably inclined Eskimos, " strangers
are usually regarded with more or less suspicion, and in
ancient times were commonly put to death." The same
situation prevailed among the American Indians. Cremony,
for example, writes that " an Apache is trained from his
earliest infancy to regard all other people as his natural
enemies." This is more or less true of the Indians in general,
and especially so of the Seri. In South America, many
tribes of the Amazon valley are so hostile to all strangers, on
whom they wage war, that very little is known about them.' [2]

The ceremonial hospitality extended to strangers by Arab
tribes and others is almost certainly to be interpreted as an

[1] Davie, op. cit., pp. 234–235.   [2] *Ibid.,* pp. 13–14.

effort to mitigate the initial hostility. An amusing transitional
case is seen among the Nigerian natives, where 'guests might
be entertained, but would be robbed or enslaved on the road
next day.'

These quotations provide us with a general picture of life
in primitive communities. What is most striking is the small
groups in which primitives live, their friendly behaviour
towards group comrades and their hatred of neighbours,
coupled with the propensity to see nothing but good in their
own group and nothing but evil in others. With this in mind
we can fruitfully discuss the occasions which provoke war and
the apparent objects of it.

Davie classifies them under four headings—war for land
and booty, for the capture of women, for cannibalism, and
wars resulting from religious motives such as the obligation of
blood revenge and human sacrifices. Of these, wars for land,
booty and women can obviously be best understood in terms
of acquisitiveness, whilst motives such as the desire for revenge
will be found to require theories of animism and projection to
explain them.

Acquisitiveness.

Land, women, booty and human flesh appear to be the
commonest requirements of primitive man. Davie gives
innumerable examples of hunting tribes resisting any trespass
on their hunting grounds, herders fighting over the possession
of water-holes and grazing grounds, agricultural communities
disputing boundaries.

> ' The encroachment of one hunting tribe on the lands of
> another was a persistent cause of hostilities among the
> American Indians, who were very jealous of their boun-
> daries. Near the mouth of the Mackenzie River, warfare
> arising from violation of tribal boundaries was incessant ;
> anyone found hunting out of his own territory was slain.
> The disputed right of the Flatheads to hunt buffalo at the
> eastern foot of the Rockies was the cause of long-continued
> hostility with the Blackfeet. Encroachment on the hunting
> grounds of other tribes was a cause of war among the
> Central Californians, the Omahas, and the tribes of
> the lower Mississipi valley and elsewhere. The wild
> tribes of the valley of Mexico " attacked all who entered
> their domain, whether for hunting, collecting fruit, or
> fighting."
> ' In Africa, especially in the south and east, a life-and-

death struggle for the possession of the water-holes and grazing grounds has led to incessant warfare with the extermination of many tribes and the forced migration and dissolution of innumerable others. The more or less civilized herders of to-day are frequently at war for similar reasons, and the historical migrations and invasions of barbaric races into Europe, Asia, and elsewhere belong in the same category. Among the Bedouins, the chief cause of war is jealousy over watering places and pastures, while grazing grounds and the right to use the streams for irrigating purposes are a fertile source of quarrels among the Berbers of Morocco.'[1]

Animals and material goods are frequently fought for. This is especially the case amongst nomads, where property is mostly portable and therefore easily stolen. Some tribes are even stated to make their entire living this way. Many illustrations could be taken from Scottish history of cattle-lifting. The blacks of Africa behave in a similar way.

'Throughout the continent, wherever cattle raising is the chief occupation, cattle lifting is the most frequent *casus belli*.

'Among the Galla and Abyssinians, who wage war for cattle, each warrior receives a certain portion of the booty, the leader getting the lion's share. By far the majority of East African wars are over cattle. The pastoral Vanika make war only to steal cattle while the chief occupation of the Masai is the same. "The Masai do not do, nor will they do any form of work whatsoever beyond tending their cattle and raiding. . . . Their whole life is spent in breeding cattle and stealing it. All fighting comes incidentally. Their greed for cattle is insatiable." They, too, are occasionally raided, however, and warriors, fully armed, guard the cattle day and night.'[2]

The raids of nomads upon agriculturalists for the produce of the soil are yet another variation of primitive battles from motives of acquisitiveness.

'The warlike Matabele of South Africa are a scourge to all the neighbouring agriculturists, as are the Sákalávas of Madagascar, who plunder the fields of the Hovas. Among the Chin Hill tribes of India, there was until quite recently a "raiding season" extending approximately from October to March, after the crops had been gathered and when there

---

[1] Davie, op. cit., pp. 78–79.   [2] *Ibid.*, pp. 84–85.

was no work of great importance to be done in the fields. It was then that the hillmen perpetrated atrocities in the plains, kept the tea-planters of Assam on the alert, and almost annihilated the wretched border subjects of the king of Ava. Similarly the Koiari, who inhabit the mountains of the interior of New Guinea, " go down to the coast occasionally for the purpose of robbing the plantations of the Motu " ; and the people of Tatana, near Port Moresby, who have no plantations, live by plundering those who have.'[1]

In the more advanced peoples who have learned the value of labour the desire for slaves is a powerful motive in going to war. ' From time immemorial the Africans have enslaved one another and have been enslaved by other peoples. . . . For centuries European traders and shippers aggravated the condition of slavery already existing in Africa by promoting wars and raids for the sake of human merchandise, and more recently their role has been taken over by the Arabs. Throughout the continent slavery rivals cattle-lifting as the chief cause of war.'[2] War for slaves also existed amongst some of the Naga tribes of India, a few of the Indians of North and South America, in New Guinea and the Solomon Islands.

The desire for women is another cause of acquisitive wars. The Maoris have a proverb : ' Land and women are the roots of war.' Like most proverbs it is a half-truth. It leaves out of account motives arising from religious and superstitious beliefs which, in some communities, are of vital importance. Yet disputes over land are frequent amongst primitives and as was intimated in a previous section, the desire for females is a frequent source of conflict amongst men as amongst baboons.

In many parts of the world woman capture has been a regular custom and has naturally resulted in as regular warfare. Amongst certain tribes, in fact, it is said to have been the principal cause of war.

' Among the Ba-Huana, women constitute one of the chief causes of war, and the frequent wars of the Ba-Yaka arise principally from charges of adultery. It has been said of the Boloki that "ninety per cent of their quarrels were about women, for every man who had one or more wives bitterly resented any interference with his sole proprietorship in them." Almost all the quarrels of the Nigerian tribes are over women, and the capture of women is one of the

[1] Davie, op. cit., pp. 87-88.   [2] Ibid., pp. 90-91.

chief causes of war. Among the Fang, " the chief causes of war are disputes over women and these feuds may last for years. Owing to a bitter feud it is often impossible for the women to work in the gardens or fish on the river, the consequence being a great scarcity of food." This situation is due to the fact that the Fang make no distinction of sex in their fights, shooting down women as well as men. Bennett, who reports the above facts, says that in Foulabifong, where he resided, " a woman palaver (dispute) lasted over ten months, and the three adjoining towns were in a state of famine "—a clear demonstration of the economic importance of women.'[1]

Similar statements are made about tribes in the Pacific Islands and amongst the American Indians.

There can thus be no doubt that the desire to capture women leads to war, but it is a little surprising to find anthropologists differing over the motives which lead to woman capture. Davie argues, in opposition to Letourneau, that the gratification of sex-passion ' is quite secondary to the economic motive.' It may be true that primitive men desire women as workers and slaves, but it is at least open to doubt whether this is his main object in stealing them. Taking into account our knowledge of human nature and of baboon behaviour, we are inclined to adopt the Frenchman's hypothesis. But the question can only be solved satisfactorily by a closer examination of available evidence.

The desire for human flesh is also stated to be a cause of war, but it is difficult to know to what extent it really is so. There can be no doubt that many primitive tribes eat their prisoners and also those slain in battle, but this is different from starting a battle in order to obtain meat for the larder. Davie asserts, however, that cannibalism is ' commonly prompted either by actual want or by a liking for human flesh ' and quotes much evidence from Melanesia and from Africa in support of his view. Some of the Congo tribes are said to have regarded human flesh as a special delicacy—' it is very nice and better than any other meat '—and others cured the bodies of the slain as we cure bacon. The Miranhas of South America regarded human flesh as a ' rare, dainty meal.'

But there are other motives for eating your enemy besides hunger and *gourmandise*. One is the aim of destroying the enemy entirely, another that of submitting him to the utmost

---

[1] Davie, op. cit., p. 98.

indignity and so gaining revenge.[1] Again primitives hold the view that the man who eats his enemy will acquire his virtues. But it is obvious that these motives are not really *causal* of warfare. You do not want to destroy an enemy until you have got one and the explanation of why neighbours are regarded as enemies is further to seek.

The foregoing evidence demonstrates abundantly that acquisitiveness is often a cause of war. Land, food, women, slaves are desired and war undertaken for their capture. But these requirements are not to be thought of as arising simply from the struggle for existence. Primitives are no more solely concerned with the bare requirements of a livelihood than civilized beings. Their desire for prestige and their competitive valuation of possessions are of great importance. Many possessions are of no real use but are coveted simply as marks of wealth and rank. An instance is the value set upon the intersexual pigs in the New Hebrides. They cannot breed, are not eaten, nor are they used for any other purpose. Yet they are much sought after and their owners deemed worthy of respect. The prestige value of cattle in Africa is also of great importance, altogether apart from food value.

' It is said of the Bahima of Africa that " they form warm attachments for the animals ; some of them they love like children, pet and talk to them, coax them, and weep over their ailments ; should a favourite die their grief is extreme, and cases are not unknown in which men have committed suicide on the loss of a favourite animal." . . . Cattle have a similar hold on the imagination of the Bechuana. Their possession assures social position. A common saying is : " The person who has no cattle is nothing at all of a person." Cattle are not merely the chief wealth of these people ; they are even regarded as the clan-gods of their fathers.'[2]

These instances remind us of the way children value anything which other children want, and demonstrate that the desire for land and booty even amongst primitives is by no means explained simply by their need for food.

The psychology of possessiveness is extremely complicated. Biological urges, such as the needs of nutrition and reproduction, undoubtedly play an important part in many of man's

---

[1] An even greater indignity is to leave the dead man in the oven or to tell a prisoner : ' You are not even worth cooking.' Even to-day in Fiji it is a most appalling threat to exclaim : ' Were it not for the Government, I would eat you.' (Davie.)

[2] Davie, op. cit., p. 83.

acquisitive activities. But they rarely play the whole part, and in some they seem hardly to appear at all. In many parts of the world, for instance, men go to war simply for the purpose of capturing victims for human sacrifice ; others prey upon their neighbours for no other reason than to obtain their heads. There is no conceivable biological nor economic explanation for such practices. Biology and economics fail also to explain the very numerous wars which result from the widespread tendency for one tribe to make a scapegoat of its neighbour. For an understanding of such wars, which there are grounds for believing are more numerous than any other kind, we must enlist the aid of psychology, particularly the psychology of animism and projection.

Animism and Projection.

The custom of blood-revenge leads to many primitive communities living in a state of perpetual warfare with their neighbours. Revenge for another man's death appears a simple enough motive at first sight. But on examination problems arise. For instance it may be asked why it is that two peoples should keep up age-long vendettas which are manifestly to their mutual disadvantage, and why they cannot come to some arrangement and live together on friendly terms. Again it is not obvious why tribes divide up their neighbours into friends and foes. If a comrade is killed by a member of a friendly tribe an amicable settlement is arranged and no feud results, whereas a similar incident involving an enemy tribe will be followed by ruthless and bitter reprisals. No understanding of such a malignant state of affairs is possible without an appreciation of the deep mistrust with which rival communities view each other, a mistrust which leads to wild accusations of malevolence and does not even require a real incident, such as murder or wife-stealing, to lead to an attack. For the evidence shows that, under the influence of animism, *any* misfortune which a community suffers is immediately attributed to the malevolent hand of another, resulting, of course, in a war of revenge. Wars of revenge because of real damage done must, therefore, be regarded as more justified and intelligible instances of a deep-rooted tendency to punish your neighbour for any harm which you may suffer, whether he be really responsible for it or not.

On pages 95–97 several instances were given of primitive peoples laying the blame for disease and other natural disasters at the door of the spirits, and then demonstrating against and attacking the malevolent creatures. Exactly similar processes lead to war when, instead of spirits, neighbouring communities are incriminated.

'Between tribes or districts which are not normally friendly, warfare becomes a more serious and more deadly matter. Any misfortune which a community may suffer, be it the death of one of its members, injury to the crops through drought or flood, ill-success in fishing or hunting, or any other mishap which by Western Europeans would be regarded as due to natural causes or an " act of God," is as a rule attributed by the Melanesian to the evil machinations of a neighbouring group, and will sooner or later lead to reprisals by means of magic or force of arms.'[1]

'For instance, the Motu of south-east New Guinea have a superstitious fear of the neighbouring Koitapu, to the magical power of whom they attribute any calamity befalling them. In 1876 they lost much of their sago in a storm at sea, their frail canoes being unable to withstand the rough water and carry the cargo. They charged the Koitapu with bewitching their canoes and killed many of them in revenge. Again, in 1878 after a prolonged drought, for which they held a Koitapu village responsible, they attacked the village and killed all they could. " As the drought had long continued, rain soon followed this murder and confirmed the natives in their superstitious belief." Another instance, illustrative of the mental reactions of primitive man, is furnished by the Quissama of Angola. Should a traveller pass through their country during a prosperous season, they look upon him as a fetish, or possessed of a spirit, but should a dearth occur, he had better escape as quickly as possible, for he is blamed for it and severely handled. In the Solomon Islands and the New Hebrides, belief in the evil eye is said to be one of the most frequent causes of war.'[2]

Blood feuds are particular examples of this general tendency. In some cases they may result from an actual murder, but more often the death which has to be avenged was due to natural causes. For it must be remembered that to the primitive mind death is *never* natural. Either it is due to evil spirits or else to the magic and witchcraft of nasty neighbours. Should a man have the misfortune to be eaten by a crocodile whilst bathing, the crocodile is not deemed responsible, but

[1] Wedgewood, *The Causes of War in Melanesia. Oceania*, I.
[2] Davie, op. cit., p. 115.

the man or spirit who by magic caused the crocodile to be hungry. If a man is smitten by disease, it is the enemy who sent the disease who is to blame.

' The tribes of Assam, for instance, hold that illness and death are caused by an evil spirit projected by some member of a hostile tribe. The supposed magician or witch is commonly put to death. If he is a member of another tribe, war between the two groups may result.'

' Belief in witchcraft is a fruitful source of war in Polynesia. It leads to similar results in New Guinea. Not long ago part of the Toaripi tribe left Eavara to settle nearer the coast. Soon after the settlement was formed, a large number of tribesmen developed a bad form of ulcerated legs. It was decided that they were the victims of sorcerers, who were supposed to be members of the faction which had opposed leaving Eavara. A quarrel ensued and developed into a tribal fight. The Kiwai Papuans are frequently incited to war by similar beliefs. About 1890, for example, a party of Sumai natives went to Domori where they were treated hospitably, but shortly after their return home one of the leaders of the party became ill and died. His spirit, it was held, appeared and reported that a certain Domori man was the cause of his death. His tribesmen thereupon attacked Domori and killed several of its inhabitants.'[1]

Numerous similar examples could be quoted from Australia. ' Spencer and Gillen say that under normal conditions in Central Australia, every death means the killing of another individual. If the alleged sorcerer is a member of some other tribe, an avenging party starts out and war ensues.'[2] A similar state of affairs was common amongst the Indians of both North and South America.

No simple psychology of possessiveness or revenge can explain these facts. Moreover, as Wedgewood points out, many even of the more rational incidents which lead to war, such as the stealing of women or disputes over fishing or garden rights, are only ' the necessary sparks which fire the train of hatred and suspicion which ever lies between the two peoples.' This irrational and all-pervasive suspicion, which insists that even natural calamities be attributed to others' evil machinations, the authors regard as of paramount importance in any understanding of war. It is this suspicion which magnifies trivial incidents to gigantic proportions, leads to

[1] Davie, op. cit., p. 116.   [2] *Ibid.*

feelings of insecurity and, finally, to outbursts of aggression. Modern Europe demonstrates it quite as plainly as Oceania. We must, therefore, ask what is the cause of such irrational suspicion and hatred.

The role of animism is obvious. Nothing is the result of natural forces ; a human agent is behind everything. But animism does not explain why someone *outside* the group is so regularly incriminated. This, in the authors' submission, is only to be understood as being the result of the projection of condemned impulses on to outsiders ; the group as a whole, probably led by a medicine man, regarding itself as innocent and others as guilty.

It has already been shown that this is a general tendency of groups. They exalt themselves and regard everyone else as ' bad people ', capable of any kind of witchcraft. Once begun the tendency to attribute all evil to your neighbour grows like a snowball and leads to constant fear and hatred. Moreover, since the projection is mutual, each group tends to make a scapegoat of the other. It thus appears that the Melanesian habit of ' beating up ' a neighbouring island is only a special instance of the very widespread custom of attacking with intent to destroy some scapegoat who is made responsible for every disaster. When spirits are made the scapegoats, a war on the spirits is the result ; when it is another human community, war on that community ensues.

It is perhaps worth emphasizing that the terror lest they themselves are responsible for these disasters is plainly discernible in the beliefs and practices of most primitive tribes. For instance, when a relative dies the savage immediately fears that the dead man's ghost will return to torment him. The universal fear of recently dead ghosts and the precautions which are taken to keep them away seem to us clear indication that the relatives are afraid that they will be held responsible for the death. Frazer[1] has dealt with this subject at length.

' The general attitude of primitive man to ghosts, even of his own kinsfolk, is one of fear, and far from attempting to retain them in the dwelling or to facilitate their return, he is at great pains to drive them away, to keep them at a distance, and to bar the house against their unwelcome intrusions. The means to which he resorts for the sake of thus keeping the spirits of the dead at bay are very various, and often display an ingenuity and resourcefulness worthy of a better cause.'

[1] Frazer, *The Fear of the Dead in Primitive Religion.*

' Among the Alfoors of Minahassa in Northern Celebes, when a wife has died before her husband, the widower is led by a woman, with his head muffled, from the house to the place where his marriage was celebrated, there to take a last farewell from his departed spouse. The children and nearest relations follow, lamenting. Arrived at the place, *the woman beseeches the spirit of the dead wife to go away and not to come and trouble the widower and children and make them ashamed.*'

' The Karieng are the aboriginal inhabitants of Siam, who, when the Siamese or Thai invaded the country from the north, retreated to the mountains on the east and west where they still remain. They burn their dead, after which they detach a bone from the skull and hang it on a tree, together with the clothes, ornaments, and weapons of the deceased. After performing dances and pantomimes, accompanied by mournful songs, some of the elders carry away the bone and the belongings of the departed and bury them secretly at the foot of a distant mountain, begging the ghost not to return and torment his family, since everything that he owned has been buried with him.'[1]

The dead man is always conceived of as being in a rage with his erstwhile friends. It is hardly surprising that they, therefore, do their utmost to foist the blame on to someone else and to sacrifice them to appease his wrath. Thus blood-revenge is seen to have much in common with human sacrifice, which is also undertaken to appease an angry spirit and which also frequently leads to war. The differences are that sacrifice is more formalized than revenge and implies an admission of guilt. The god to whom the sacrifice is made is closely connected with the spirits of the tribe's ancestors, but he is usually not a man recently dead. Moreover, sacrifices are made on other occasions besides death, for instance in the event of epidemics or famines.

It is interesting to note that these natural disasters can appear to a people in two guises. In Melanesia they seem commonly to be interpreted as the mischief wrought by *bad* neighbours on a good people. In more advanced civilization they appear as punishments sent by an angry and *righteous* god, sitting in judgment on a sinful people. Although this question needs far fuller analysis than is possible here, it seems to us that these two attitudes can be roughly interpreted as resulting in the first instance from a projection of bad impulses,

---

[1] Frazer, op. cit., pp. 33, 170, 172–173 (our italics).

and in the second from a projection of a punishing and retaliatory super-ego.[1]

The projection of bad impulses on to your neighbours has already been seen to lead to ' beating up ' expeditions. The projection of a punishing super-ego on to a god also leads to war, but in a rather different way. The epidemic or drought or defeat in battle, whatever it may be, is interpreted as punishment meted out by an angry god on to his sinful people. To stop the punishments the god must be propitiated, and this takes the form of slaughtering criminals or prisoners of war as sacrifices. Westermarck has described it as a ' method of life-insurance'. The many are saved by the sacrifice of a few, the scapegoats. And when there are not enough suitable prisoners to hand, wars are undertaken to collect them. The result is therefore the same. In both cases a neighbour is made to bear the sin. Many instances where human sacrifice has led to aggression and war are quoted by Davie.

For instance,

' The Batjwapong of South Africa, whenever there was a drought, would waylay a man and strangle him, hoping thereby to appease the gods and secure rain.'

' In Benin, terrible human sacrifices were an integral part of the religious ceremonies and rites, especially when an enemy was at the gates. The yearly sacrifices numbered thousands, and to secure the requisite victims the King of Benin would send out his army to raid other villages.'

' Among the Mayas of Central America, captives, if of noble birth, were sacrificed to the gods, especially at the great feast of victory ; prisoners of plebeian blood were offered only in default of victims of higher rank. Raids were also occasionally undertaken with no other object than to obtain victims.'[2]

The annual sacrifices seem to be simply the payment of a regular premium to keep the god sweet. They are the preventive side of religion as against the curative roles of particular sacrifices in situations of emergency.

---

[1] Although, in the authors' view, the fear that a god is angry is the result of a projection of a severe super-ego on to the Deity, it should be noted that this is not the same thing as saying that the idea of God is nothing but the projection of the super-ego. In our view psycho-analysis has added little to our knowledge of whether a God exists or not. What it has done has been to demonstrate beyond doubt that man's conception of the Deity is heavily distorted by processes of projection.

[2] Davie, op. cit., pp. 133–135.

Yet another instance of wars resulting from the fear of the malevolence of neighbours are head-hunting expeditions. Although acquisitiveness run riot plays a large part, the underlying motive appears to be the fear that merely killing your neighbour is insufficient. His spirit remains vengeful and therefore dangerous. Since the soul is believed to reside in the head, by capturing the head you gain possession and therefore power over the soul. If you are nice to the spirit and propitiate it, the plagues, pestilence and murder, over which he has control, can be averted.

'A tradition among the Kenyahs of Borneo stated that a frog told them to cut off the heads of their enemies instead of merely the hair, which had formerly been taken to decorate their shields, because "if you were to take away the whole skull you would have everything you required—a good harvest and no sickness, and but very little trouble of any kind." When Furness asked a Kalamantan native why they killed one another for their heads, the latter replied : "The custom is not horrible. It is an ancient custom, a good, beneficent custom, bequeathed to us by our fathers and our fathers' fathers ; it brings us blessings, plentiful harvests, and keeps off sickness and pains. Those who were once our enemies, hereby become our guardians, our friends, our benefactors." '[1]

Methods of greasing the palms of the captured spirits vary from feasts in their honour down to the offering of cigarettes.
The wars resulting from these beliefs have been numerous and devastating. Davie gives details of tribes which have been completely wiped out by the head-hunting expeditions of neighbours, and of others who live in complete isolation and constant preparedness because of it.

.   .   .   .

The examples quoted demonstrate beyond doubt that psychological processes such as animism and projection play a part in the wars of primitives, and go far to confirm the psycho-analytic theory of war advanced by Glover.[2] Sceptics may be inclined to enquire, however, whether their rôle is of any vital importance, whether they are not merely trimmings to a fundamental economic motive. It is, of course, always easy to pick material to prove any thesis, but we do not feel that the material here presented is particularly speciously selected. Our chief source has been Davie, whose suppositions

[1] Davie, op. cit., pp. 138–139.   [2] Glover, *War, Sadism, and Pacifism.*

ı

and conclusions are heavily biassed towards regarding war as the result of the struggle for existence. Again and again he writes of war as arising from the vital biological need of food.[1]

Moreover categorical statements by field anthropologists testify that economic motives, such as the desire for land, are often of minor importance in causing war compared to motives of revenge arising from a belief in animism.

There is Kingsley's statement that ‘ the belief in witchcraft is the cause of more African deaths than anything else. It has killed and still kills more men and women than the slave-trade.’[2]   Simson states that amongst the Laparo Indians in South America the belief that deaths are due to the sorceries of neighbours forms the basis for *most* of their disagreements and quarrels.[3]

Somerville states that in the Solomon Islands and the New Hebrides belief in the evil eye is one of the most frequent causes of war.[4]

Curr says of the Australians in general that the belief in sorcery by an alien tribesman as the cause of death is by far the most common and most serious cause of war.[5]

Finally, Lloyd Warner analysed the causes of war in the Murngin tribe.[6]

‘ For the last twenty years, out of some seventy battles that were recorded for this paper in which members of the Murngin factions were killed, fifty were caused by the desire to avenge the killing of a relative, usually a clansman, by members of another clan (blood revenge). (Of these, fifteen were killings that were done deliberately, against the tradition of what is fair cause for a war, because it was felt that their enemies had killed the wrong people when they retaliated for injuries done them.)   Ten killings were done to members of a clan stealing a woman, or obtaining a woman who belonged to another clan, by illegal means.

---

[1] The following statement may be quoted to demonstrate Davie's views :
‘ But the most fundamental cause of war is hunger or the economic motive, and it ties war up straightway with the competition of life. Groups come violently into conflict in carrying on their struggles for existence ; they fight over hunting and grazing grounds, for food, for watering places, for plunder ’ (p. 66).
It has already been remarked that Davie regards both cannibalism and the capture of women as springing essentially from an economic motive : ‘ The most elemental economic motive is the quest for food. On the lowest stages of societal evolution, men themselves are regarded as part of the food supply.   Human flesh is animal meat, and cannibalism in such cases is part of the group's self maintenance ’ (p. 66).
[2] Quoted by Davie, op. cit., p. 116.   [3] Davie, op. cit., p. 117.
[4] Davie, op. cit., p. 115.   [5] Davie, op. cit., p. 116.
[6] Lloyd Warner, *Murngin Warfare. Oceania*, II.

Five men were killed because they had slain men by black magic. The clans of the men killed by magic slew the men who were supposed to be the magicians. Five men were slain because they⁻ looked at a totemic emblem under improper circumstances and by so doing insulted the members of the clan to whom it belonged as well as endangered the latter's spiritual strength.'

It is interesting that in the wars of this tribe economic motives such as the need for food or land played no part during twenty years. But it is by no means our intention to deny the economic origins of some wars. For instance, even in Melanesia where wars are usually the result of a desire to avenge deaths and disasters by punishing neighbours, the acquisition of land has been known to be a cause. ' War undertaken for the purpose of territorial conquests such as are familiar in our own history, and as occur⁻ in parts of Africa, are relatively rare in Melanesia, and even the acquisition of land as an incident of war is not common. This is doubtless due to the fact that in most of the islands there is no serious dearth of cultivable land. That such wars do sometimes occur, however, seem certain, for there is evidence that in some of the coastal regions of Aitape district, New Guinea, the desire for a more extensive territory has been the cause of tribal conflicts. Among the Polynesian people of Tikopia there was, several generations ago, a war between the four principal groups in that island, for the acquisition of good garden land which is by no means abundant for the population which it sustains.'[1]

The truth is that primitive tribes are so numerous and their customs so different that it is only after an exceedingly careful and thorough study that anyone would be in a position to generalize about the origins of war in primitive societies as a whole. But the evidence presented by Davie, who certainly has not selected it with an anti-economic bias, makes any predominantly economic theory of warfare untenable. It leaves no doubt that psychological forces such as displacement and projection, resulting from feelings of guilt, and the belief in animism are at least as important as economic motives. Even acquisitiveness is seen on examination to be by no means synonymous with the struggle for existence.

[1] Wedgewood, op. cit.

Conclusions.

The evidence presented, we submit, allows for the following conclusions :

(1) Man in his primitive state is fully as warlike as civilized man.   In unorganized peoples feuds and quarrels are the rule, whilst organized tribes are usually in a state of constant warfare with their neighbours.

(2) Peace within a tribe seems to be bought at the expense of continual warfare without.   This we have explained as being due to the displacement of any hostile feelings which may be aroused against friends on to ' foreigners '.

(3) Apart from this general motive for fighting neighbours, two others can be discerned—possessiveness and the need for a scapegoat.

(4) Possessiveness is not a simple motive and cannot be identified with the struggle for existence.   In addition to economic motives such as the desire for land, food, and slaves, wars are waged for the capture of women and of ' useless ' booty.

(5) The need to find a scapegoat leads to widespread war. The scapegoat motive has been shown to lie behind the constant mutual suspicion in which many communities live, a suspicion which leads to an outbreak of hostilities and wars of revenge upon the least provocation.   When the provocation is purely imaginary, as when crops fail, the scapegoat theme is obvious ; when real provocation occurs, for instance over murder or wife-stealing, it is the scapegoat motive which leads to general warfare and prevents a pacific solution.   The raids for procuring sacrificial victims are also prompted by the necessity to find a scapegoat, in this case a ceremonial one.

(6) No evaluation of the relative importance of these motives is possible without more thorough investigation.

(2) WAR BETWEEN CIVILIZED COMMUNITIES

It is impossible to deal adequately with the warlike motives of modern States without elaborate historical and sociological research.   This we have not attempted, partly because we have little experience in this field and partly because the relevant material is contained in such a vast and scattered literature that the time required to sift it is prohibitive. We have consequently confined ourselves to a discussion of such motives as irrational acquisitiveness and the need to find and expel scapegoats as they appear in modern life.   Although we believe that these forces are usually grossly underestimated, we do not feel that we are in any position to assess their true social influence relative to other factors, as for instance the rational acquisitive or economic motive. It is to be hoped that the research necessary to make such an estimate will soon be undertaken.

Acquisitiveness is no doubt of great importance in impelling modern nations to aggression. This may sometimes have a solid economic motive such, for instance, as the desire for the gold and diamond mines which prompted Great Britain to the South African War. But the interest in possessions is not simply economic any more than the Kaffir's interest in cattle is solely for their food value. For instance, until the recent German claim for colonies, many Englishmen took no interest in their colonial possessions. But immediately someone else wanted them, these people become possessive whilst at the same time maintaining that colonies are of no use to anyone.

The point which, in our view, requires emphasis is that the strength of the possessive feeling with its accompanying potentiality to aggression is, even in civilized peoples, not proportionate to the real economic or political advantages involved. In adults, as with children, possessions are possessions, and will be fought over with a violence only partially dependent on their real value. Of course there is always an attempt to justify covetousness on biological or economic grounds and it is consequently difficult to persuade people that other motives play a part. It would lead us too far into the psychology of possessiveness to deal with this question adequately, but one factor can be touched upon.

It will be remembered that both baboons and children were observed to fight more for the possession of their comrades than of material things. Baboons fight for the possession of females, children for the attention of parents and other grown-ups, primitive man for the possession of wives. Civilized man, on the other hand, rarely proclaims that he is fighting for personal possessions. Usually he maintains that he fights for material economic gain when he fights for possessions at all. But this claim does not always bear close examination. Material property, such as land, jewellery and even food, is often found on investigation to be a substitute for, and to symbolize, a person. The desire for the possession of the person and their affection has been transformed into the desire for the possession of certain inanimate property. Such a process is shown in its crudest form by the fetichist, who will obtain sexual satisfaction from the possession of some article of clothing. But such symbolization is not confined to the fetichist. There is no one who does not place especial value upon an object because of its personal associations, be it a flower ' worth ' twopence or a diamond ' worth ' two hundred pounds. The article comes to symbolize the person who gave it and its value becomes the value of their affection.

Sometimes the symbolic value remains of subsidiary importance, but at other times it plays the major part. The latter is occasionally demonstrated by thieves. A friend tells how her mother employed a servant girl who was an orphan and had been brought up in an institution. After a while it was found that articles disappeared and the girl's room was searched. In her drawers were found, in addition to a few articles of female finery, a large collection of photographs of her employer's family. Clearly what the girl most wanted were family relations and the affection which she had never had.

Motives of this type, we believe, underlie much of the irrational attitude of civilized man towards his possessions. Parnell, describing the Irish Nationalist Movement which had for its main objective the rescue of Ireland from the foreign English, remarked : ' You would never have got young men to sacrifice themselves for so unlucky a country as Ireland, only that they pictured her as a woman. That is what makes the risks worth taking.'[1] The idea of a ' motherland ' is, of course, a common one, but the implications of the symbolism are not usually recognized. For what it implies and what Parnell implied is that *the combative feelings aroused are appropriate, not to the narrow economic value of the land in question, but to the value of the person whom it is symbolizing* (in this case an idealized mother).

In the evaluation of an object, the ' real ' economic value and the personal symbolic value are always intertwined. Both are important, sometimes the one predominating, sometimes the other. An analysis of their inter-relations is an essential preliminary to an understanding of possessiveness, and this we hope to carry further in a later work.

Besides acquisitiveness, in both its rational and irrational aspects, there is another primitive force which in our view plays a major rôle in shaping the relations of modern states to each other. This is the *scapegoat* motive. It has already been shown to play a large part both in individual aggressiveness and also in the wars of the simpler peoples. Here we hope to show that it is exploited no less relentlessly by civilized States.

[1] Haslip, *Parnell.*

An increase of civilization seems to do little to mitigate the the craving for someone upon whom all misfortunes can be blamed. Science has only served to discredit the magical and superhuman agencies held responsible by primitives. We no longer look for the sources of all evil in the spirit world as savages do. A man of culture and science is too enlightened to believe even in witches or the devil. But the need for a scapegoat remains and has to be satisfied, and, since supernatural beings are no longer available, it is members of other races, religions and political creeds who are incriminated. To the Fascist, the Communist or the Jew is at the root of national degradation and economic distress, to the Communist it is the Fascist or the Capitalist who is engineering his slavery. Therefore each persecutes the other with an undying zeal, like members of rival Christian sects in the past.

Sometimes it is difficult to detect the presence of the scapegoat motive. If often lurks behind charges which have an objective basis, or is insinuated so subtly that it beguiles the unwary. But there is at least one nation which makes no mystery of its need for a scapegoat and who proclaims the scapegoat's sins in such fantastic terms that the aid of a psycho-analyst is not required to detect the underlying motive. Indeed the leaders of Nazi Germany have provided in their speeches and writings about Jews and Bolshevists and in their own accounts of numerous pogroms a permanent and ineffaceable record of witch-hunting in twentieth-century Europe.

Ever since the war, the National Socialist movement in Germany has been preaching the wickedness of Jews and the absolute necessity for their expulsion if Germany is ever to regain her old position in the world. The result has been widespread persecution and social violence amounting almost to civil war. More recently the identification of Jews and Bolsheviks has turned this hatred from the internal enemy, the German Jews, to an external enemy, the U.S.S.R. An examination of the Nazi literature inciting the people to fight either Jew or Bolshevik, with the consequences of domestic persecution or fierce international hatred, seems to us to throw much light upon the sources of mass violence.

We shall begin by comparing the Nazi attitude to Jews with primitive man's attitude towards evil spirits and neighbours.

The failure of crops or of hunting and fishing expeditions is put down by the Melanesians to the evil machinations of their neighbours. To the Nazi, economic depression is due to the Jew. Dr. Goebbels ' after declaiming that " they need not think we shall let the Jews depart unhindered if the crisis becomes serious," went on to say that "the hatred and fury and desperation of the German people would then turn against those who are reachable in the country." '1

The natives of Queensland attribute rape to a 'noxious being called Molonga.' The Nazi incriminates the Jew. 'This Jew is forced by his blood to ruin and to decompose all other races. He is driven by his blood and by his inborn abnormal sensuality to ravish non-Jewish women and girls.'2 'Moreover, the Jew has in his veins a large element of negro blood ; his frizzy hair, his wolf lips, the colour of his eyeballs, prove this as effectually as the insatiable sexual greed which hesitates at no crime and finds its supremest triumph in the brutal defilement of women of another race. This bestial lust obsesses even a barely mature Jew boy. . . .'3 Hitler himself says as much in his book : 'The black-haired Jewish youth lies in wait for hours, satanic joy in his face, for the unsuspecting girl, whom he defiles with his blood and thereby robs from her own race. . . . There were and are Jews who brought negroes to the Rhine, always with the same aim and idea in their minds of destroying, through the bastardization that must inevitably result, the white race which they hate—of bringing it down from its high cultural and political level and themselves getting the mastery over it. . . .'4

On the Gold Coast of West Africa, epidemics are attributed to evil spirits. Hitler makes the Jews responsible for venereal disease. Jewish doctors in Germany, instead of curing disease, are held by Holtz to inject a 'specifically alien poisonous substance into the German blood.' 'We should have fought and died in vain,' he writes, 'if we were to leave the Jew his greatest domain for robbing and murdering the German people, if we were to leave him medicine.'5

No savage in any land can die unless it be by the black magic of his neighbour. No Nazi can die without its being the work of a Jew.

'In Tauroggen, a Memel district, a maid killed her illegitimate child and was arrested. The National Socialist

1 *The Times.*
2 Quoted from *Der Stürmer*, October 1931, by E. A. Mowrer in *Germany puts the Clock Back.*
3 Quoted from *Der Stürmer* in *The Yellow Spot : The Extermination of the Jews in Germany.*
4 Adolf Hitler, *Mein Kampf*, German edition, p. 357.
5 Leading article in *German Health from Blood and Soil* (February 1935) by Karl Holtz, editor of *Der Stürmer*. (Quoted in *The Yellow Spot*, p. 148.)

official organ in Königsberg, *The Preussische Zeitung*, immediately spread throughout Eastern Prussia the story that this was ritual murder. As a result Jewish shops were destroyed and pilfered in several towns, including Allenstein. A month later the Berliners were told this story as a ritual murder. *The Judenkenner* said :

' " Year out, year in, in every corner of the earth, from country districts and in towns, both old and young disappear. Some of these are snatched away by the Jews so that they may spice the devilish meal of their thirty to forty millions, and enable them secretly and criminally to revel in the idea that, like that of those poor stupid victims, they will one day suck the blood of the whole of mankind when once they have stupefied it sufficiently." '[1]

Jews were responsible also for the World War. ' The Jew . . . gave birth to this hatred and cherished it until the very day when the Tsar was induced to sign the order for mobilization. . . . Tsarism was to be overthrown in order that the Jewry of Russia might snatch equal rights, nay—privileges.'[2] ' The most frightful ritual murder that the world has ever seen was to be perpetrated ; the Aryanry of the world, the flower of mankind, was to be rooted out. This was the will of pan-Jewry, and these were the commands of the Jewish Kahal.'[3]
They have been behind every political death in Germany since the war.

' Herr Hitler, in the course of his oration, said that the nations had to tread painful paths in order to find salvation. The milestones were invariably graves, in which the best of their manhood lay. From the days of the Red November revolution, those who had devoted themselves to the cause of Germany, who had stood for a new and better companionship of the people, and at no time harmed any man, had been menaced by a sinister supra-national power.
' In the severe fighting of the first three months of 1919 German men fell everywhere, shot down by the bullets of their countrymen. They did not die because they had any hatred of those countrymen, but only because of their love of Germany. Behind this madness they saw everywhere

---

[1] *The Yellow Spot*, p. 57.
[2] Hitler's Speech : ' World Jewry and the World Stock Exchanges, the Real Culprits in the World War,' 13 April 1924. (Quoted in *The Yellow Spot*.)
[3] Ritual murder number of *Der Stürmer*. (Quoted in *The Yellow Spot*.)

the same power, everywhere the same apparition which led these men and goaded them and finally put the pistol or dagger into their hands. He referred also to the murder of Thule associations in Munich, and said that the originators were again the members of this sinister power which was and is responsible for this fratricide in their nation. *He most solemnly declared that on the path trodden by the National Socialist Movement there lay no single opponent who had been murdered by them, not even an attempted assassination, but an endless row of murdered National Socialists* almost always foully struck down from behind. Behind every murder stood the power responsible for that of Gustloff; *behind the harmless little German incited to the deed stood the hate-filled power of their Jewish enemy ; an enemy which they had never sought to harm, but which had tried to subdue and enslave the German people, and which was responsible for all the misfortunes that had haunted Germany through the years.*[1]

This was a funeral oration for a Nazi who had been assassinated in Switzerland in February 1936. On reading it, it should be borne in mind that it was about eighteen months after 30 June 1934, when hundreds of Nazis were murdered on Hitler's orders by members of their own party.

Primitives are less vocal than Nazis, so that some of the Nazi accusations against the Jews cannot be paralleled. For instance, Hitler proclaims that ' in culture the Jew defiles art, literature, and the theatre, destroys natural sentiments, undermines all ideas of beauty and dignity, of nobility and goodness, and drags humanity down under the spell of his own base mode of life.' . . . ' When the Jew wins political power he casts aside the few wrappings which he still has. The democratic Jew of the people becomes the Jew of blood and tyranny. He tries in a few years to root out the national carriers of intelligence, and by robbing the peoples of their natural intellectual leadership, prepares them for their lot as slaves in permanent subjection.'[2]

Finally a convenient summary of Jewish crimes may be found in the following National Socialist leaflet.[3]

---

[1] *The Times*, Feb. 1936. (Our italics.)
[2] *Mein Kampf*, German edition, p. 358.
[3] Translation of a leaflet reproduced in *The Basler Nationalzeitung* of 25 September 1935. Reprinted facsimile in *The Yellow Spot*, p. 198.

FELLOW GERMAN,
  do you know :
  that the *Jew*

ravishes	your child
defiles	your wife
defiles	your sister
defiles	your sweetheart
murders	your parents
steals	your goods
insults	your honour
ridicules	your customs
ruins	your church
corrupts	your culture
contaminates	your race

  that the *Jew*

slanders	you
cheats	you
robs	you
regards	you as cattle

  that *Jewish*
  doctors murder you slowly
  lawyers never try to get you your rights
  provision shops sell you rotten foodstuffs
  butchers' shops are filthier than pigsties

FELLOW GERMANS, DEMAND THEREFORE :
  etc. etc.

So much for their writings. What of their acts? The persecution of German Jews by National Socialists now belongs to history. Whilst violence and bloodshed were widespread in the early days of the Nazi regime, legal persecution no less vindictive, though perhaps less dramatic, remains the rule. Jews are excluded from all civil rights, from the civil and military services and from many professions. They are not permitted to teach, in some towns they may not even use the trams. The evil spirits have been expelled.

The Germans' own descriptions of some of these expulsions bear a curious resemblance to anthropologists' records of similar rituals in other lands.

For instance : ' When an epidemic is raging on the Gold Coast of West Africa, the people will sometimes turn out, armed with clubs and torches, to drive the evil spirits away. At a given signal the whole population begin with frightful yells to beat in every corner of the houses, then rush like mad into the streets waving torches and striking frantically in the empty air. The uproar goes on till somebody reports that the cowed and daunted demons have made good their escape by a gate of the town or village ; the people stream out after them, pursue them for some distance into the forest, and warn them never to return.'[1]

The Nazi celebrations hardly differ except in the amount of human suffering inflicted.

' On Thursday at 5 p.m. the swastika flag was hoisted on the property of the last Jew to leave Hersbruck. The Hersbruck district is now definitely purged of Jews. With pride and satisfaction the population takes cognisance of this fact, recognizing that this " spring cleaning " is first and foremost due to District Party Leader Comrade Sperber, who has emphasized the Jewish danger at thousands of meetings, until the people realized the truth and the last Jew left the district. . . . We are firmly convinced that other districts will soon follow suit and that the day is not now far off when the whole of Franconia will be rid of Jews, just as one day that day must dawn when throughout the whole of Germany there will no longer be one single Jew.'[2]

These quotations leave no doubt that the persecution of the Jews in Germany is prompted by the same motive as impels the primitive to persecute the spirits or his neighbours. The objects of persecution in each case are held responsible for everything, real and fantastic, about which the people feel guilty. No doubt many other motives come into play in the actual selection of victims for persecution. Personal spite and professional jealousy have played their part. But it is clear that the main form of the campaign is only to be understood in terms of scapegoat psychology. However, this conclusion does not explain why the need for a scapegoat has overwhelmed Germany during the past fifteen years. It is true that most people have the need to a greater or less extent all the time, but experience shows that it usually requires a great disaster to stimulate it to such a pitch that it takes complete possession of a person or a people. What is it then which has recently made Germany have such desperate need of a scapegoat that they have believed and acted upon these insane accusations against Jews ? Fortunately there is no mystery about it. Hitler has explained it at length in his book.[3]

[1] Frazer, *Golden Bough*, p. 550.
[2] Reported in the *Fränkische Tageszeitung* on 26 May 1934 and quoted in *The Yellow Spot*, p. 89.
[3] Hitler, *My Struggle*. Authorized English translation. Chapters VII, X, XI.

The German collapse of November 1918 came upon Hitler, the front-line soldier, as a crushing blow. Honourable defeat he might have borne, but a defeat brought about by internal disruption made him mad with shame. Describing his feelings upon hearing the news of revolution and capitulation he writes :

' Was the Germany of the past worth less than we thought ? Had she no obligation owing to her own history ? Were we worthy to clothe ourselves in the glory of the past ? In what light could this act be presented for justification to future generations ?

' Miserable depraved criminals !

' The more I tried in that hour to get clear ideas about that tremendous event the more did I blush with burning rage and shame. What was all the pain of my eyes in comparison with this misery ?

' There were horrible days and worse nights to follow. I knew that all was lost. In those nights my hatred arose against the originators of that act.

' The Emperor William had been the first German Emperor to offer the hand of friendship to the leaders of Marxism, little guessing that scoundrels are without honour. Whilst they held the Imperial hand in theirs, their other hand was already feeling for the dagger.

' With Jews there is no bargaining—there is merely the hard " either—or."

' I resolved to become a politician.'

He is immediately overcome by dreadful feelings of unworthiness and guilt,[1] feelings which gradually develop into the conviction that Germany's defeat was a punishment which she had fully deserved.

' Germany's military defeat was, alas, not an undeserved catastrophe, but a merited chastisement of eternal retribution. The defeat was more than deserved by us.'

' . . . the military collapse was itself but the consequence of a series of unhealthy manifestations and of those who proposed them ; they had already been infecting the nation in times of peace. The defeat was the first visible catastrophic result of a moral poisoning, a weakening of the will

[1] It is always interesting to speculate on the psychology of dictators, though available evidence confines us to tentative suggestions. There seems reason to believe that Hitler felt intense guilt over his mother's death and that the defeat of Germany in 1918 was regarded by him as a repetition of her death. In his book he describes how, when he learnt of the defeat and the proclamation of the Republic, he wept for the first time since he had stood by the grave of his mother.

to self-preservation and of doctrines which had begun many years previously to undermine the foundations of nation and Reich.'

His analysis of the origins of this ' moral poisoning ' follows.

' If we divide the human race into three categories— founders, maintainers, and destroyers of culture—the Aryan stock alone can be considered as representing the first category.'

The Aryan is the only creative race and all other civiliza- tions have followed from his beneficent rule over other peoples. But unfortunately the Aryan has not always maintained racial purity with the result that civilizations sometimes crumble and have to be built afresh. ' Blood-mixture, and the lowering of the racial level which accompanies it, are the one and only cause why old civilizations disappear. It is not lost wars which ruin mankind, but loss of the powers of resistance, which belong to purity of blood alone.'

This poisoning of the Aryan blood is due to inter-marriage, in Germany's case with the Jew, who is naturally barbarian and can only suck culture from others. ' The exact opposite of the Aryan is the Jew. . . . Thus since the Jew never possessed a culture of his own, the bases of his intellectual activity have always been supplied by others. His intellect has in all periods been developed by contact with surrounding civiliza- tions. Never the opposite.' ' The Jew . . . was ever a parasite in the bodies of other nations. . . . His propagation of himself throughout the world is a typical phenomenon with all parasites ! He is always looking for fresh feeding grounds for his race.'

There follows the familiar description of a Jewish plot to gain control of Germany, to ' destroy the elementary principles of all human culture,' and ' to tear down all which may be regarded as the prop of a nation's independence, civilization, and economic autonomy.' This leads to his conclusion.

' Thus, if we review all the causes of the German collapse, the final and decisive one is seen to be the failure to realize the racial problem and, more especially, the Jewish menace.

' The defeats on the field of battle of August 1918 might have been borne with the utmost ease. It was not they which overthrew us ; what overthrew us was the force which prepared for those defeats by robbing the nation of all political and moral instinct and strength by schemes which had been under way for many decades ; and only these instincts can fit nations for existence and justify them in existing. By ignoring the question of maintaining the racial basis of our nationality, the old Empire disregarded the one and only law which makes life possible on this earth.

' The loss of racial purity ruins the fortunes of a race for ever ; it continues to sink lower and lower in mankind, and its consequences can never be expelled again from body and mind. . . . . .

' That is why, in August 1914, a nation did not rush full of determination into the battle ; it was merely the last flicker of a national instinct of self-preservation face to face with the advancing forces of Marxism and pacifism, crippling the body of our nation. But since in those fateful days no one realized the domestic foe, resistance was all in vain, and Providence chose not to reward the victorious sword, but followed the law of eternal retribution.'

The reasoning is typical of its kind. The national calamity, defeat, was sent as a punishment for the sins of the nation. Those sins must therefore be expiated if further disasters are to be avoided. Accordingly Hitler ordained that the Jews should be sacrificed to purge the nation of moral corruption, just as many primitive peoples have ordered the murder of hundreds of thousands of criminals, prisoners of war or slaves, in the belief that this would free them of their sins and make their god less angry.

' At Onitsha, on the Niger, two human beings used to be annually sacrificed to take away the sins of the land. The victims were purchased by public subscription. All persons who, during the past year, had fallen into gross sins, such as incendiarism, theft, adultery, witchcraft, and so forth, were expected to contribute twenty-eight ngugas, or a little over two pounds. The money thus collected was taken into the interior of the country and expended in the purchase of two sickly persons " to be offered as a sacrifice for all these abominable crimes—one for the land and one for the river." A man from a neighbouring town was hired to put them to death. On 27 February 1858 the Rev. J. C. Taylor witnessed the sacrifice of one of these victims. The sufferer was a woman, about nineteen or twenty years of age. They dragged her alive along the ground, face downwards, from the King's house to the river, a distance of two miles, the crowds who accompanied her crying :   " Wickedness ! Wickedness ! " The intention was " to take away the iniquities of the land. The body was dragged along in a merciless manner, as if the weight of all their wickedness was thus carried away." '1

It seems remarkable, almost incredible, that a great modern nation should be swayed and overwhelmed by such primitive motives. But the written word of the Nazis' own prophet leaves no other interpretation possible. Defeat was felt as a punishment for sin. The avenging gods demanded a sacrifice and the Jews were picked as the victims. By this means the Germans were enabled first to admit the guilt they clearly felt and then to free themselves of it. Germany was guilty—yes—guilty of moral corruption and selfishness. But the guilt did not belong to true Aryan Germans, it belonged solely to the Jews and could therefore be remedied by the simple expedient of expelling them.

This idea of defeat and revolution as a national disgrace, the cause of which must be foisted upon someone else, is met again and again in Nazi literature. ' When Jews made their revolution in Germany a new slaughter of human beings began. Whoever resisted the November criminals had to die. Both citizens and peasants.'2 (In actual fact, of course, the revolution began in the German Navy.) ' The Jew is the cause and beneficiary of our national slavery. He ruined our race, rotted our morals, hollowed out our way of life, and broke our strength.'3

But if the defeat of 1918 gave birth to National Socialism, the economic slump of 1931 nurtured it and brought it to power. Without this further calamity, with its corresponding load of guilt which had to be shifted on to other shoulders, it is doubtful whether Germany would ever have reached explosive point. As Goebbels points out, the more serious the crisis became, the more violent grew the hatred and fury of the German people. Despite the fact that no one could legitimately be blamed for the world-wide disaster, the conviction that someone is responsible for everything demanded that the culprit be found and retaliation inflicted. Such an atmosphere naturally favoured an extremist party, one, moreover, which had already fixed the blame for everything upon the Jews. The result was the 1933 election in which Hitler obtained political power with the consequences already described.

---

[1] Frazer, *Golden Bough,* p. 569.
[2] Quoted in the *Yellow Spot* from the Ritual Murder Number of *Der Stürmer.*
[3] Quoted by Mowrer, op. cit., ' from an oft-reprinted National Socialist proclamation.'

Now it will be seen that the authors' analysis of Hitler's rise to power with the accompanying flood of hatred and bloodshed lays little emphasis on simple economic motives, such for instance as envy of the positions held by Jews in the professions and trade of the country. Economic jealousy may have contributed to the result, but no economic theories can explain the extraordinary charges brought against the Jews, nor explain the similarity of the German pogrom to the witch-hunting of medieval Europe or the persecution of spirits by primitive tribes. In our view the forces which make for rage and violence are the same in all these instances, the belief in animism, the fear of guilt, and the need to find a scapegoat. Simple economic motives are almost as out of place in the explanation of the Jewish persecutions in Germany as they are in explaining the violence with which the natives of the Gold Coast drive off the cholera demons.

But because the persecution of Jews was demonstrably irrational, this does not mean that it was politically useless. On the contrary, the subsequent feelings of relief and emancipation have been very real, as real as the feelings of depression and futility that had been prevalent before. Germany has lost much in the process. Many good citizens and able men have left her shores and the respect of decent citizens in other countries has been forfeited. But she has released herself from a sense of inferiority and guilt and regained self-confidence and that most precious of all beliefs, that she is a good nation capable of adding to civilization, blameless of its destruction. By blackening the Jews, Nazis have been enabled to indulge in comforting fantasies of their own goodness and rightness and to persuade themselves that they are not bad, dangerous people. Goebbels, in one of his self-righteous speeches, announces : ' All we National-Socialists are convinced that we are right, and we cannot bear with any one who maintains that he is right. For either, if he is right, he must be a National Socialist, or, if he is not a National-Socialist, then he is not right.'[1]

This sense of absolute rightness, a certain indication of repudiated feelings of guilt, is often carried by Hitler to the borders of megalomania. Of the ' Jewish doctrine of Marxism ' he writes :

' It would, therefore, as a principle of the Universe, conduce to an end of all order conceivable to mankind. And as in that great discernible organism nothing but chaos

---

[1] *The Times*, 6 October 1935.

K

could result from the application of such a law, so on this earth would ruin be the only result for its inhabitants.

' If the Jew, with the help of his Marxian creed, conquers the nations of this world, his crown will be the funeral wreath of the human race, and the planet will drive through the ether once again empty of mankind as it did millions of years ago.

' Eternal nature takes inexorable revenge on any usurpation of her realm.

' *Thus did I now believe that I must act in the sense of the Almighty Creator : by defending myself against the Jews I am doing the Lord's work.*'[1]

Similar views have often been expressed. The following are those of a certain Dr. Schreber, who also wrote an autobiography, which he named *Memoirs of a Neurotic.*

' It was, moreover, perfectly natural that from the human standpoint (which was the one by which at that time I was chiefly governed) I should regard Professor Flechsig or his soul as my only true enemy—and that I should look upon God Almighty as my ally. I merely fancied that He was in great straits as regards Professor Flechsig, and consequently felt myself bound to support Him by every conceivable means, even to the length of sacrificing myself.'[2]

Dr. Schreber's book would have been more aptly named *The Memoirs of a Psychotic*, for he was a patient in an asylum for many years suffering from delusional insanity.

. . . .

The result of attributing a nation's troubles to fellow-citizens is internal dissension, leading, perhaps, to civil war. The result of incriminating another State is international hatred and the danger of international war. The attitude of Nazi Germany towards Bolshevist Russia illustrates this.

Of recent years much of the Nazi hatred hitherto mobilized against the Jews has been diverted against Bolshevism and all the same fantastic charges repeated. Actually the one scapegoat has been transformed into the other by the neat device of identifying the two. This identification was already made in Hitler's book, but it was not fully developed until the Nuremberg Congress of 1936—' The Congress of Honour '—where Jew and Bolshevik became interchangeable terms. Whilst Hitler only referred occasionally to the ' Bolshevik

---

[1] *My Struggle*, pp. 35–36. (Our italics.)
[2] Quoted by Freud, *Collected Papers III*, p. 398.

Jews' and the 'Jewish-Bolshevik Soviets,' his Minister for Propaganda, Dr. Goebbels, expounded their identity at length.[1]

'Bolshevism is a pathological and criminal madness clearly originating from Jewish sources and led by Jews with the object of annihilating European civilization and the attainment of an international Jewish world domination over it. . . .'

'Jews made the Bolshevik revolution in Russia, but the original revolutionary clique had been practically exterminated and Jewry remained the leading influence. Thus every internal Bolshevik quarrel was more or less a Jewish family affair, just as the latest executions in Moscow were nothing but one gang of Jews shooting another in the pursuit of power. It was wrong to suppose that the Jews were necessarily united. They were only united when they found themselves in a minority threatened by a preponderant national majority. Once in power the old quarrels broke out again.

'The Bolshevik idea, the unscrupulous destruction of culture and civilization with the fiendish aim of annihilating the people, could only originate in a Jewish brain, however much they might seek to hide the fact in Western Europe. Germany alone in Europe has had the courage to denounce them for the criminals they were. Once upon a time in Germany men were imprisoned for pointing out a Jew as a Jew. The Nazis did it then nevertheless, but the world still refused to allow it. Nevertheless, they believed that as they had been able to convince the German people of this danger, so they would eventually succeed in opening the eyes of the world and showing it Bolshevism in its true colours. And meanwhile they would not weary, through all the fearful crises assailing so many nations, in telling the people again and again of the unholy danger which threatened them and in calling to them : " The Jews are to blame ! The Jews are to blame ! "

'In fact, Bolshevism is the foulest tyranny of blood and terror that the world has seen. Jews conceived it and to make their rule impregnable Jews are carrying it out to-day.'

It is difficult to believe that a Cabinet Minister can speak of a neighbouring power in such terms. 'The Bolshevik idea, the unscrupulous destruction of culture and civilization with the fiendish aim of annihilating the people. . . .' That

[1] Speech at Nuremburg, 10 September 1936.

is a phrase which might be expected from a grandiose lunatic suffering from delusions of persecution, but is hardly credible from the mouth of one of the leaders of a great European power. Yet it is no isolated exception. At the same conference Dr. Rosenberg speaks of the ' gangster millions ' of the Soviet which ' spread destruction throughout the world, a bitter challenge to all who still value their culture and civilization ', whilst Herr Hess elaborates the villainies of Bolshevism in Spain, concluding : ' What human brains can conceive in the way of cruelty is being given reality. In Spain Bolshevism is displaying itself in its stark infamy. In Spain Bolshevism is giving renewed proof that it is a mockery of civilization,' and Hitler himself proclaims Bolshevism as the universal enemy of Europe.[1]

' And we are appalled by the thought that some of the democratic countries may be unable, as they develop, to find a natural and characteristic spiritual form, but may fall a prey to Bolshevism, our hatred of which comes of a natural repulsion for that menacing, aggressive and bestial doctrine.'

(Herr Hitler then continued the now-familiar diatribe against Bolshevism. It had first joined issue with National Socialism by invading Germany with its Marxist theories, just as it now endeavours to threaten them by bringing its military force nearer to their frontiers, since the first plan had failed.)

' We were successful in attacking, destroying, and blotting out Bolshevism in our internal politics : and now, since we know that these attempts to meddle with our internal affairs still continue, we are obliged to declare Bolshevism the deadly foe in our external affairs, and to recognize the equally great danger which comes from its constant approach. We have fought Bolshevism in Germany as a power which tried to poison and destroy our people : and we will fight it as a world power when it endeavours to bring the Spanish disaster, with new and more violent methods to Germany. And we will not be led aside by the chatter of those weaklings who only believe a danger when they are swallowed up by it.

' But the object of Bolshevism is not to release the people from their afflictions, but, on the contrary, to extinguish the healthiest, soundest elements, and put in their place all that is most corrupt. I can make no pact with a doctrine whose first act on obtaining power was not to liberate the

---

[1] Speech at conclusion of Nuremburg Congress, 13 September 1936.

working masses, but to release from the prisons the concentrated anti-social scum of humanity, in order then to release these monsters on a terrified and distracted world.'

The internal enemy has become the external enemy. Instead of a Jewish evil within, which is destroying culture, rotting morals, and undermining the State, Hitler now views a Bolshevik danger coming from Russia, intent on poisoning and annihilating the German people. And just as he threatened to destroy and expel the Jews when his chance came, so does he threaten Bolshevism. It is true that there is no direct hint of invading Russia. Rather does he envisage a defensive war against a rapacious and bestial assault. But the need and desire to annihilate the focus of Bolshevik infection is clear throughout.

'We can therefore afford to observe these subversive attempts on the part of others (i.e. Bolshevists) with a certain calm. Should, however, the Reich ever be threatened by such an attempt the nation would, as one man, remember the National-Socialist watchword, and in a sweeping rush expel those who thought that their task would be more easily achieved by military means than by the doctrinal methods of recent years. In these days of international revolution, let them take note of this : in Germany the German people is going to be master in its own house, and it will not have any Jewish-Bolshevik Soviets.

'I am watching the course of Bolshevik infection of the world to-day just as carefully as I did years ago when I saw this infection in our people and warned them against it. I see the methods of Bolshevik corruption of the peoples and I see their preparations for the great upheaval. It is my ardent desire that it may be given to our movement in Germany to solve in peaceful work the great problems set it. They are tasks to be undertaken in a spirit of high endeavour, and I know that their completion will perpetuate not only my name but above all the name of our movement in Germany.

'But let Bolshevism, which a few months ago we heard was increasing its military strength with the intention of starting a revolution, and, if necessary, *forcing the gates of other countries*,[1] let this Bolshevism realize that before the German Gates there stands a new German army ! '

Goebbels also warned Russia :[2]

'The Red East threatened, but the Leader was on guard.

[1] Our italics. Compare German invasion of Austria, March 1938.
[2] Nuremburg, 1936.

Germany, as the outpost of European culture, was ready and determined to repel this danger with every means from her frontiers. The Bolshevik pest in Germany had been exterminated, and it would find no further opportunity of raising its head. Should Moscow attempt to revive Communism in Germany they would be met with ruthlessness which would surprise even the Bolshevik rulers. The Party was the guardian of international peace, and the army, as the defender of the country, constituted a shield under which the nation could feel safe.'

Nazi Germany, the all-good, has become the hero defending the fair maid of Europe from the vicious and dangerous dragon of Bolshevism.

This pose as a world saviour is a sure indication that the mechanism of projection is working full-blast. In the eyes of Hitler and Goebbels the Aryan is perfect—he has no sin—and all the evil in the world is due to the presence of Jews and Bolsheviks. Our conclusion that these accusations spring from the need to ease uneasy consciences is confirmed by various passages from their speeches. For instance, by dwelling upon the enormities of Bolshevist political measures (which we do not dispute) Hitler is able to paint National-Socialist methods in colours rather rosier than their records justify.

'National Socialism, therefore, presents a serried front against Bolshevism on racial grounds, and in the interests of the German people and of the German worker. We reject this doctrine also on account of our more humane methods towards our fellow-men. The statement of the speaker at this congress and events in Spain have given the world and our fellow-citizens in Germany an insight into the atrocities of Bolshevik methods of fighting and maxims of government. The German people is too good and too honourable for such hideosities.

'We National-Socialists have also a revolution behind us ! That revolution also was made by workers, peasants, and soldiers. It also defeated an enemy and cast him to the ground. But it is a proud thought for us that, when in January 1933 the National-Socialist revolution swept over Germany, not even a window-pane was broken, that we were able to defeat murderous plots, and even the numberless cowardly assassinations of our followers committed by the Communists, with the minimum of defence and no retaliation at all. Not because we were too weak to see blood—we endured the most terrible suffering of human history as soldiers in the hardest war of all time, at a moment when the leaders of Bolshevism were running round Switzerland as cowardly *émigrés* or making their gain as unnatural profiteers in Germany and in Russia. We led our revolution as we did, and not otherwise, because it is repugnant to us to inflict more suffering on people just because they are our political opponents than is inevitably necessary for the secure defence of our regime. Every civil war brings suffering, but most of all those in which poor working men are incited to run into the face of machine-gun fire, while their Jewish leaders know well how to find a safe way, at the decisive moment, to their carefully invested futures abroad.'

Bolshevik methods of fighting, and maxims of government are full of atrocities. Contrast the German people ! They are too good and too honourable for such hideosities ! When the Nazis came to power, not a window-pane was broken and there was no retaliation at all ! The projection is obvious and it is obvious too in the following specific accusations which, amongst many more general ones, Goebbels levels at Russia.[1]

'We National-Socialists are honest enough to allow our rule of the people to be reaffirmed almost yearly by a general secret ballot. Bolshevism prates of the people, of the land, of peasants, and workmen, but *its real character is nothing but force.*'

.   .   .   .

'It was the achievement of the Soviet Union to have literally reintroduced slavery. About six and a half million men had gone through hell upon earth in the *forced labour camps* of Bolshevik Russia. Hundreds of thousands of corpses strew the Stalin White Sea Canal, built by forced labour under the leadership of Jews in the G.P.U.'

.   .   .   .

'Bolshevism, while claiming to have saved the peasantry from disaster, had, in fact, driven them to hunger and want. *It constantly oppressed them by the system of police espionage.* The summit of this oppression was the law of 7 August 1932, punishing the peasants with death or ten years' imprisonment for every misdemeanour ; in the application of this law they even used children to inform against their parents.'

.   .   .   .

[1] Speech at Nuremburg, 10 September 1936. (Our italics.)

' *Despite these tremendous armaments Bolshevik propaganda pretended that Moscow is pursuing a policy of peace and has no desire for expansion or aggression.*'

It is typical that Goebbels should indict Bolshevist Russia for the very same practices for which Nazi Germany has become famous.

Finally we may quote rather a curious passage from one of the Führer's speeches[1] which suggests that he has some insight into himself.

' The fact that people cannot see a thing does not mean that it does not exist. For years in Germany I was laughed at as a false prophet. For years my admonitions and predictions were regarded as the visions of a man suffering from mental disease. This was said by those worthy *bourgeois* who had no use for the Bolsheviks in their own business and therefore stoutly refused to believe in the existence of the danger. *Because these dull-witted fellows, owing to their very mentality, naturally had no leanings towards Communism they would not envisage such awful possibilities in others.*'

It seems that only people with an inclination towards Communist atrocities can envisage such awful propensities in others. We are inclined to agree, for clinical work has confirmed over and over again that only people with rapacious and savage impulses are inclined to see them in their neighbours.

These examples make it clear that in at least one Western power the tendency to find a scapegoat to blame and persecute for all the national troubles is no whit less powerful than it is in so-called primitive peoples. Many other examples of a war-like attitude engendered by the scapegoat motive could be given but perhaps none so naked and unashamed.

No doubt it is easier to see the way in which foreigners make scapegoats than it is for us to recognize the same tendency in our own nation. Democracies perhaps make less use of foreign countries and races as their scapegoats than do totalitarian States, for the very reason that in a democracy there is always a rival political faction to blame for all the troubles which beset the country. For instance, many Conservatives are convinced that the Labour administration of 1929–1931 was responsible for the economic crisis, whilst most Socialists would put it down to Capitalists and bankers. Both projection and animism play leading parts in this mutual recrimination. For the man-in-the-street it is just as difficult

[1] Nuremburg, 13 September 1936. (Our italics.)

to believe that economic depression is due to impersonal economic forces over which we have as yet no control as it is for the natives of the Gold Coast to conceive of an epidemic except as the work of a malignant devil. To blame foreigners or any special group of fellow-countrymen as responsible for the slump is just as fanciful as to blame a devil for cholera, and perhaps more dangerous. For little harm comes from the violent expulsion of imaginary spirits or from sending a wretched goat to die in the wilderness as the Jews used to do. When you have expelled the demons you may live in dread of their return, but at least other men remain your friends. But to persecute men is to make dangerous enemies who may revenge themselves on you. Ceremonial demonstrations against an evil spirit held responsible for unemployment would be preferable in very many ways to irresponsible campaigns against this or that political party, race or nation.

The foregoing analysis of some modern manifestations of mass violence has demonstrated that irrational greed and ' righteous ' indignation springing from a repudiated sense of guilt play their parts. It is not possible to examine their relations to each other at any length, but it is worth observing that they often, perhaps usually, march hand in hand, the one justifying the other. Sometimes, when the main motive to war is avarice, the projection of evil on to others is undertaken in order to justify the greed. But at other times almost the opposite seems to be true. It would seem probable that the main driving force in some European wars, as in Melanesian, is the desire to destroy a scapegoat, and that this is disguised as a necessity for economic expansion. In other words we suggest that economic motives are as often used to justify scapegoat-hunting as is moral condemnation of the enemy to justify greed.

This brings us to the question of what motives actually prompt individuals to take part in a war. They are probably very varied. Displacement of aggression from friends to foreigners and the hope of promotion and success no doubt play a part, but the delight in finding a public scapegoat against whom all our friends are prepared to fight seems to us all-important. Many who fought for England in 1914 must have felt better men because Germany could be painted so black, and they could see themselves as the saviours of all that is good. For psycho-analytic investigation has demonstrated that the scapegoat motive is operative, if not in everyone, at least in the great majority. In some the demand for a scapegoat is constant, in others it remains dormant, appearing whenever guilt is increased by sad events, others' criticism or a propagandist campaign. It is the latent propensity in each individual towards creating scapegoats which a popular leader works upon. This is illustrated by the course of events in Germany since the War. Very many Germans in 1918–1919 must have felt as Hitler did, burning with shame and humiliation that they should have been defeated. And just as Hitler immediately looked round for a scapegoat to expel, so must thousands of other Germans. Thus the defeat enormously increased the potential demand for a scapegoat, just as in Melanesia it is raised after a storm or a famine. The chief difference between a leader and his followers in this situation is that the leader has a more pressing need to find a scapegoat and an almost abnormal determination to lay the hounds on his tracks. In Germany the Führer made the demand for a scapegoat vocal, he pointed the quarry and incited the pack. But he could not have been successful had not his harangues against the Jews and Marxists met with a response from the hearts of the German people. They too had need of a scapegoat, less vocal, perhaps less violent than their neurotic leader's, but none the less insistent. In our view it is this half-conscious, undirected, popular demand which provides the energy for a political scapegoat campaign, which can be awakened and directed but never manufactured by its leader. Hitler, the prince of propagandists, has a clear understanding of these springs of popular mass action and has never ceased to exploit them.

' Men do not die for business, but for ideals.
' Nothing displayed the Englishman's psychological superiority in readiness of a national ideal better than the reasons he put forward for fighting. Whilst we fought for daily bread, England fought for " freedom "—not her own, but that of the little nations. In Germany they mocked at this effrontery and got angry, proving thereby how thoughtless and stupid Germany's so-called Statecraft had become before the War. We had not the slightest conception of the nature of the forces which could lead men to their death of their own free will and volition.'

.   .   .   .

' This was realized by the British propaganda with very real genius. In England there were no half statements which might have given rise to doubts.
' The proof of their brilliant understanding of the primitiveness of sentiment in the mass of the people lay in the

publication of horrors, which suited this condition and both cleverly and ruthlessly prepared the ground for moral solidity at the front even when great defeats came along, and further, in nailing down the German enemy as being the sole cause of the War. . . . . .'[1]

'Men do not die for business, but for ideals,' and the desire to destroy those upon whom they have projected all their own wicked impulses. It is because so few are free of a latent need to see and fight their own bad impulses in others that popular movements incriminating a party, race or nation are able to carry even sensible men off their feet, to instil into them beliefs which in their sane moments they would know are ridiculous and impel them to actions of which in other circumstances they would be ashamed. It is the latent need for a scapegoat in every one of us to which such movements as anti-Semitism or anti-Fascism appeal and which accounts for the self-righteous enthusiasm which carries so many good men away when war is declared. In our view it is only by recognizing and controlling these irrational sources of hatred and greed that society can be purged of war. Since dealing with such problems in the individual is the daily task of the psychotherapist, it seems that he should be able to point the way by which society might hope to handle their mass manifestations. But the application of individual methods to social problems is highly complicated, and we feel that, for the present, diagnosis is all we can attempt. In a later work we hope to suggest a cure.

Conclusions.

In this fragmentary attempt to analyse the causes of hatred and violence in civilized societies, the following tentative conclusions have been suggested :

(1) Working hand in glove with rational acquisitiveness (the economic motive) are the forces of irrational acquisitiveness. The value of land and other property as symbolizing people is stressed and such terms as ' motherland ' taken seriously. The aggression aroused in disputes over property is appropriate not merely to the economic value of the property but to the value of the person whom it symbolizes.

(2) The need of a scapegoat is believed to play as large a part in civilized communities as it does in primitive. The causes of the persecution of German Jews are shown to be of a

[1] *My Struggle.* pp, 70 and 83.

similar nature to the causes of the expulsion of devils by primitives. The differences lie not so much in origin of hatred as in the victims selected. Exactly the same motives are held to be at the root of certain international hatreds. The hatred of Nazi Germany for Bolshevik Russia is instanced and analysed.

(3) Propaganda is successful only in so far as there is a potential need for a scapegoat in the populace. In leaders this need is more pressing and more vocal, but it is impossible to account for the hatred which can so easily be stimulated in ordinary citizens in certain circumstances without supposing that there is this need latent in everyone.

J. B.

INDEX